CW00516818

Caro Giles

Twelve
Moons

**Harper
North**

HarperNorth
Windmill Green
Mount Street
Manchester M2 3NX

A division of
HarperCollins*Publishers*
1 London Bridge Street
London SE1 9GF

www.harpercollins.co.uk

HarperCollins*Publishers*
Macken House,
39/40 Mayor Street Upper,
Dublin 1, D01 C9W8

First published by HarperNorth in 2023

1 3 5 7 9 10 8 6 4 2

Copyright © Caro Giles 2023

Caro Giles asserts the moral right to
be identified as the author of this work

A catalogue record for this book
is available from the British Library

HB ISBN: 978-0-00-854323-5

Printed and bound in Great Britain by
CPI Group (UK) Ltd, Croydon

All rights reserved. No part of this publication may be
reproduced, stored in a retrieval system, or transmitted,
in any form or by any means, electronic, mechanical,
photocopying, recording or otherwise, without the prior
permission of the publishers.

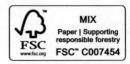

This book is produced from independently certified FSC™ paper
to ensure responsible forest management.

For more information visit: www.harpercollins.co.uk/green

For anyone feeling small under dark skies

Contents

A note on moons

The moon has inspired and guided us from our earliest origins. Part of an eagle's wing was discovered in a cave in the Dordogne Valley, marked with notches in a serpentine pattern, suggesting an interest in lunar cycles as early as the Palaeolithic period. Twelve pits set in a curving arc in a Scottish field are said to form one of the oldest lunar calendars in the world, dating back 10,000 years. And still we stare up at the sky.

The word 'moon' can be traced to the Old English 'mona', as well as being linked to an Indo-European root meaning month, and the Latin 'metiri' or measure, since the moon measures time for us. Yet it is also timeless because we have never known life without it, and its cycles offer a sense of return and renewal. The moon continues to intrigue cultures, faiths and communities across the world, connecting us to the seasons and often named accordingly. These names are spoken in every tongue, from indigenous American languages to Gaelic, Hindi to Chinese.

The titles of the chapters in this book are taken from a combination of Celtic, Medieval, Anglo-Saxon and Old

English names, woven as they are to the hills and beaches explored in this story. Although the names generally allude to the full moon, in this book they refer to the moon in all of its phases. Some alternative descriptors from these cultures are also listed, though there are many, many more.

Whatever name we use, we all breathe under the same moon.

1
Wolf Moon

Stay Home Moon, Moon After Yule,
Quiet Moon

She is dancing in front of the window. Twisting, skipping and curling her hands as if they will conjure a spell. The light outside shines blue on the rooftops, still covered in yesterday's ice. Steam is floating up from heat vents, like witches' breath.

The sky is clear: sharp and brittle with the cold air, and stars prick the black like a spindle, blurring in her stare. The heat from the girl's eyes could match the energy of those stars, so fierce is the kick in her heel, the snap of her long hair. The moon hangs steady and pregnant with hope, only days away from completion. Hours earlier it was a tissue paper wish invading the sunlit day, translucent and hesitant. The girl pounds her bare feet on the floor, child cheeks flushed and smooth. She is dancing for the Wolf Moon.

* * *

The first full moon of the year must, by necessity, break open the sky with its lustre, and offer hope of a better future. This year, the world is exhausted and broken, perhaps more than anyone remembers. Diseased and dysfunctional, humans desperate to avoid unwittingly killing the ones they love have been forced into isolation by a deadly virus. A little country floating in the North Sea is cut off from the rest of the world, after gorging on its own ego.

Amidst this chaos, I light candles while my children sleep. I look out of my window over the rooftops of a Northumbrian market town and imagine the sea beyond, watching as the sky appears behind the houses as a thin strip, sometimes ripping the world apart in bright oranges and pinks, other times creeping in on a cloud.

I dream and I worry and I sip my tea, and somehow the darkness soothes me, this mother who has birthed four daughters, and must now raise them in a world that has revealed itself to be harsh and relentless. I worry about how I can show them magic and calm, when they have already seen cruel and unfair, and I tilt my head from side to side, feeling the tension of life creaking. And all the time the darkness is there, a cloak around my aching shoulders, and the candles dance.

In these hours when the world is sleeping, I feel invincible. I am a mother of course, but I am also the promise of my own future, of who I can become. As I sit and watch the shadows cast from the candles, I see myself dancing, skirt spinning, hair caught in the wind, and I know that a better version of me is emerging. This new version feels fear just like before, but I am trying to become more aware of myself and my own needs, learning that I am allowed to cling to my truth, that my voice holds value. And it is in this act of waking early and sitting in darkness that these thoughts grow stronger, so that they hold me steady when the sun is stark and bright, and there is nowhere to hide.

One January morning, rain falls, heavy and relentless in the black. I rise early, feeling the burn of tiredness and yesterday's tears in my eyes. Wrapping my dressing gown around my creaky body, I pad downstairs to the light of my mobile phone so as not to wake the children. Flicking the switch on the kettle, I lean against the worktop as the cat curls around my legs. A pipe cleaner lies in the middle of a kitchen floor that will later reverberate with the sound of bouncy hoppers and shouting girls. I pour biscuits into a plastic bowl for the cat, who chews a few noisily, then stands hopefully at the door. I know that the cat will regret running down the little path where raindrops are bouncing off the stone - she will cower beneath a car as the water trickles down the road and wait to be let back in. But she must find this out for herself and I must make my tea, so I watch the tail disappear predictably under the car and return to my kettle.

There is something soothing about the soft pressing of the teabag against the side of the mug, squeezing gently so that the leaves do not escape and swim into the boiling

3

water. My mind wanders to the demands of the day and I quickly finish making the tea and go back upstairs to my candles, hoping they will stave off reality for a little longer.

There are candles all over the house: on window sills, next to the fireplace, inside oil burners, on the desk. The reassurance that has grown from the act of lighting the wicks and watching the wax melt into liquid means that I will sometimes carefully place a candle into my shopping trolley, just in case, company for the times when darkness oversteps the mark. This morning I am burning a large, circular three-wick candle bought as a present at Christmas by my eldest daughter, The Mermaid. For a few moments the liquid makes a heart-shaped pool. But only fleetingly.

It is unlikely, I think, as I gaze out of the window, that even the moon, with all of its power, will show itself tonight. The raindrops feel like a symphony of tears, a lament for all of the pain. I want to garner the strength of the full moon: the last few years have been some of the most helpless in my life. But I have read somewhere that it is common to feel disconnected and emotional at this point in the moon's cycle, and that knowledge makes me feel less alone. It feels helpful to shed some of the responsibility and cast it into the sky.

I sit at my desk, tucked into a corner on the landing and I type, wondering if the act of turning tapped keys into words on a screen will write me back onto the page. As I type and sip my tea, the rooftops slowly start to emerge as a familiar silhouette. There are no award-wining sunrises today and already I am missing my cloak of darkness. I wonder if a lightness of spirit will come with the lengthening of the days, and what will replace the comfort of the flickering flames on my desk.

Water is dripping noisily onto the corner of the plastic roof of my utility room. It slopes on one side and the rain gathers there in a pool. When I go in there to use the washing machine, or collect reusable shopping bags, or find the hoover, or empty the litter tray, or do any of the many domestic tasks that punctuate my day, there will be a little puddle on the floor, but I don't know how to stem the leak.

It is nearly time to wake the children now and, though it is still not quite light, my mind is starting to drift towards school and shopping and no bread in the cupboard for toast. I lean over the candles, momentarily feeling their warmth on my face and, with more of a sigh than a blow, I extinguish the flames.

The new year starts as fresh as any other, like a child's face scrubbed clean with a flannel: shining and full of promise. I have followed the rules. I have sorted a pile of books next to my bed, a combination of novels and non-fiction that will nourish both the brain and the soul. I have committed to a month of decaffeinated tea and sober living. A friend has told me that drinking a pint of water as soon as I wake will change my life, and suggests that I drink it warm to make it more palatable. My

Christmas present candles are sitting patiently on my desk, waiting to be lit in a precious early morning ritual. I sign up to a challenge to run 75 miles in January, knowing that the pounding of feet on the street will provide a welcome drumbeat to accompany the rhythm of life. I sort through my children's clothes, pack away trousers that are too short for growing legs and dresses that no longer fit. They are placed into bin liners along with old books, shoes and teddies, then stacked up in piles, ready to be taken to the charity shop. I type the dates of lectures into a calendar for the online course I have recently started. Put together a timetable of virtual music lessons I will teach and somehow squeeze around the mothering and hope it will not be long before my choirs can sing together once more.

And so I am ready to face the new year. Full of intention and strength. Almost unmarried, almost free, and with a face that can still appear youthful after a good night's sleep. My eyes are large and hazel, though often I am distracted by the two little lines that furrow my brow. Hair falling in tangles down my back, or thrown into a pile on my head, long neck plaintive. Nothing is perfect.

A few short days later, wings are clipped and shutters come down. I am once more at home with four sweet daughters who can no longer attend school and need near-constant supervision. The books by the bed begin to gather dust and are replaced with Oxford Reading Tree and Harry Potter; on day fifteen I pour a glass of red wine, and feel the guilt of a nation; the pint of warm water is forgotten and replaced by steaming tea by the light of my precious candles. The utility room is full of black bin-bags that can not be dropped off because most of the shops are closed. Good intentions have fallen by the wayside when the year is still just a baby. Early mornings and running a groove in circles around my back lane are the only intentions that remain.

In the short hours bookended between the darkness, we sometimes drive to the nearest beach, where the sun hovers low on the horizon, sluggish and remote. The younger girls will run into the waves so that water soon fills their wellies and it won't be long before tiny toes begin to throb from the cold. I cover my knotty hair with an old green hat, pull it low over my eyebrows, and stare at the seaweed churning and frothing in the tide, imagining it to be a potion I could bottle up.

These trips are fleeting though, a brief tonic of air in the lungs and oystercatcher calls to sustain us through this weird claustrophobia before we must once more return to our house. A reminder that there is a world beyond our four walls, a bigger sky than the one viewed through a window frame. And a hope that by treading my feet over and over into this sand I will remember who I am, and why I am here.

* * *

On the night of the full Wolf Moon, I want to watch it rise to a fanfare of howls and steal the darkness. But the day has been one long rainstorm pouring into the dusk, sending streams splashing into gutters. The only howls to be heard are echoes from the wolves snapping at my soul.

At 9pm, I tiptoe down the stairs and slip my feet into an old pair of boots, leaving the zip undone. Pushing my arms into my jacket, I wrap a scarf around my neck, burrowing my nose into the smell of perfume and hot breath. My second daughter, The Whirlwind, the same one who danced on the landing a few nights earlier, appears from the living room and begs me to take her to find the Wolf Moon.

I had hoped to stand silent and alone, self-consciously trying to sense a shift in the night air that would announce the full moon. I want to be made to feel small under this moon, part of something huge. Often I am made to feel small by people who listen but do not hear, as if I speak a language they cannot understand. My words and actions do not always fit the narrative they are committed to, leaving me diminished and confused. When I stand and stare up at the moon, I can imagine kindred spirits doing the same, and I feel less alone. The Whirlwind is bouncing on her toes, excitement bubbling from her lips, so I tell her to grab shoes and a coat and meet me outside.

The street where we live feels Dickensian tonight. A strange, reddish smog is floating around the houses -

diffused light from the street lamps perhaps - and the air is stagnant. Although the sky is dark, I can see that cloud cover is dense and the moon is trapped. The Whirlwind is dancing around me, chattering and pointing and chasing the cat from under a parked van. There is no simmering electricity tonight, nothing special to mark the occasion. The gloomy night reflects a general malaise that currently has the world in its grip. The wolves have no appetite and there will be no howling tonight.

The terraced house we stand outside was bought by a couple who were chasing something, a fairytale perhaps. They came a little unstuck round the edges, the glue holding them together flaking and creating little gaps where the rain could get in. The man worked too hard and lost himself. The woman had many babies and wondered how she could help the man to find himself once more. The house was supposed to ground them, form a solid base on which they could build their dreams. But it was only a house, and it takes more than a mortgage to make a home.

I look up at the windows of the little house. There is one bedroom at the back and another two at the front. I now occupy the tiny one at the front of the house in a double bed I jammed between the walls because I refused to sleep in a single one. Putting aside the many children that often creep in beside me, I hold onto the possibility that I will not always sleep alone. One day I might allow someone to enter my world again and stroke my skin and maybe I won't be too scared to bare my soul.

I remember lying in another bed in the larger room at the front - the swirly white metal bed that squeaks and has a couple of broken slats. The one that my two oldest daughters now share, that is bursting with soft toys; monochrome penguins; a huge creamy dog; Piglet the hot water bottle, who used to belong to my sister. My sister doesn't need him now because she lives on the other side of the world where the sun shines hot and hard. Dressing gowns and abandoned jumpers are draped over the far end and there's a flat, warm patch where the cat likes to sleep and keep an eye on the girls.

As I stare up at the window, I am remembering a day when there was no cat and I was lying in bed with flu. It was the second year running that I had flu and I put it down to living in a constant state of stress and exhaustion. A GP friend had been to see me, and was worried about my chest, which was rattly and sore. My breathing was laboured. My friend told me I must go to the surgery, and that she would take me.

It was all I could do to climb out of my clammy pit and pull on something resembling an outfit. My bra cut into my skin like barbed wire and I just wanted to be held by someone kind. Staggering down the stairs, I was greeted by the noise of many children racing around waiting to be fed. My feet were as cold as death through my socks on the wooden floorboards.

Leaving the house felt like hell, with biting winter air nipping my feverish skin. I was bent over like a much older woman, with a coat wrapped around me, shivering and reluctant as I fell into the passenger seat. My friend pulled strings at the surgery and I was seen quickly by a doctor who told me that I was close to being sent into hospital: my chest sounded lousy and maybe there was an infection. I sat slumped and resigned in the plastic chair, not caring what was decided, because I just felt so poorly and wanted to be in my bed sleeping. In the end I was sent away, told to keep an eye on my symptoms and be in touch if they got worse, so we trundled home. I staggered up the path with dead leaves pushing against the step and shut the night behind me.

The morning after the visit to the doctor I sat in bed, chest rattling and wheezing. I cast twenty stitches onto a needle with plain black wool, and started knitting a scarf that would never be finished.

Three years later, as I stand under the absence of the Wolf Moon, I wonder if it is possible to tell a story and omit one of the main characters? Someone that looms large in my life is magnified even further by the constant dancing around him. This man was once the hero, my hero, but I no longer want him in my story.

I follow The Whirlwind back into the house now, where the air is warm and shoes scatter the hallway. *No moon tonight*, we sigh. *Let's try again tomorrow.* And when the girls are all in bed, I pull out my knitting bag, full of half-finished squares and knotted yarn. I pick up those needles again, running my fingers over the wool, surprised by how neat the stitches are. And I wonder if the wool is black because something died.

* * *

The night after the full moon, I am driving home from the city, where I have left three of my children with their dad. The Mermaid stays with me as her sisters run into his arms. Each time, as four become three, the damage spreads, like heat on silk, shrivelling everything that was once simple and beautiful. Every other Friday I pack a suitcase full of teddies, at least three for each little girl, and the blanket knitted by my grandmother for her name-sake, sucked and chewed with such love it is starting to unravel. The route is familiar now, sewn into the fabric of my life, drenched in resentment and resignation.

I point out the kestrels hovering by the side of the A1, and the North Sea to the east: either a sparkling strip of cobalt that smashes your heart or an ominous grey sliver, overhung with a fret. We sing songs that remind us of adventures we have had since our world was cleaved in two, and try to ignore the aftershocks that continue to rattle our lives. Sometimes the girls have just finished a long week of school and the youngest two, The Caulbearer and The Littlest One, are pale and exhausted in their school tracksuits. White-blonde hair frames their faces, cheeks still smooth and plump like babies.

We drive into the city. Down the slip road, over the roundabout, into suburbia and 30 mph zones indicated by tortoises on signs. Past the cancer charity that is hung with a million lights every Christmas and the red-brick houses that line the dual-carriageway. Heading into the smarter part of the city, we see a little theatre covered in pastel graffiti flowers and birds that sprawl across the grey single-storey building. It reminds me of a dream I had, with the man who is about to hold my children. A dream where all the world was a stage, a utopian Bohemia far removed from the dystopia that eventually emerged.

The dual-carriageway becomes a row of streets: at one end charity shops and a supermarket, then, as the streets become wider and tree lined, a florist, its door flanked with bay trees, and an independent school uniform store to cater for the many private school students who reside in this part of town.

As I drive here, I am wondering how it has come to this. How I have ended up on my own in the northern-most corner of England with four little girls, when I spent my childhood dreaming of bright lights and centre-stage. The little girls were definitely part of the plan, but the brutal severing of a great love was supposed to be consigned to books and theatre. I wanted to embody the epic romances I had studied, but I ignored the fact that many of them ended in tragedy.

When I left home to go to drama school, barely eighteen years old, I flitted between ashtrays and lipgloss, a child in a woman's body. High heels clattering on the pavement, a warm feeling lingering in my stomach from the free cider I had drunk using my tips jar. My flimsy white skirt was thin and short and I didn't know how lovely I was. Confident enough to show all of my arms and legs but naive enough not to understand the conse-

13

quences of naked skin. I thought I held all the power, but I didn't have a clue how to play with it.

A steady thump thump thump bounced across the road, and there was a tiny thrill from knowing the bouncer and pushing straight up the sticky, carpeted staircase. Already a little bit drunk in readiness because I was a skint student and couldn't afford club prices, I knew I'd just top up inside. Through the black swing door with a round window and scan the room. The music louder now, classic charty club stuff - *Bellissima, Encore Une Fois, Born Slippy*. In just a few years I'd be standing behind the decks of underground nightclubs in East London, but the truth is I love a cheesy tune. In two years time I would win the heart of my husband by slaying a dancefloor with *You Sexy Thing* when he said the crowd was crying out for drum and bass. A cheesy tune can make you a bride.

I would go out with a posse of bartenders who had rushed to clear tables, empty ashtrays and bottle up in time for an hour or two of mayhem before the clubs turfed everyone out onto the streets. Pubs still closed at 11, and if we were quick we could be out of the door and breathing the boozy night air by midnight. We'd spill into the room to be welcomed by regulars who needed our energy - they were mainly hammered and looking for fresh blood to inject more fun into their night. And who is more fun than a barmaid? She always puts up with the banter and gives as good as she gets. Back then I thought I was the winner. Perhaps I was just the prize.

I would chat and dab glitter on my eyes in the toilets but most of all I would dance. I'd climb behind the decks and up some steps to a cage that loomed over the centre of the dancefloor. Confident and drunk, I loved the attention. It felt like I was in charge of all the men in the room with my youth and my bare flesh and my swagger, but I was a puppet, feeling the pull of strings on my arms as I played the part expected of me. Pepsi Man, with his dark eyes and brooding stare, stood by a pillar; Dom, the pony-tailed barman, nimbly flicked bottles to rowdy lads; Chris, the cocky Mancunian with the Liam swagger, studiously ignored me and wanted me to know it. Up in the cage, I dreamt I was the fairy queen, casting them under my spell. My bleached blonde hair caught the glittery sweat on my top lip as I swung my head to the side. The balls of my feet burned as I hammered the ground in 3-inch heels, jumping and swinging in my flippy little skirt. I was a sorceress, and my watermelon Bacardi Breezer was my magic potion. This wasn't Ibiza. This was *Harpers* nightclub, Guildford, 1996.

In 1996 I was at drama school, trying to fix a broken heart by living recklessly. I felt too tall and awkward next to the petite doll-girls on my acting course and the boy I loved didn't care anymore. Drama school is a dangerous place to be when you don't know who you are. My uncle packed a couple of boxes and suitcases into the back of his estate car early one morning and drove me 300 miles south from my home in a North Yorkshire market town, to a white ex-council house in the shadow of Guildford

Cathedral. I remember my dad holding me tight and then walking briskly away so I didn't see him cry.

My three best school friends had all opted for university in Leeds, and the boy I loved, the farmer's son, the one I would do anything for, was at Birmingham University being dazzled by someone else. The gritty sprawl that was London felt like a concrete ocean between me and everything I knew, as I spread the patchwork quilt my mum had lovingly sewn for my 18th birthday over the bed in my tiny student room, and tried to think of it as home.

I want to feel that patchwork quilt wrapped around me now so I can bury my head in who I used to be and breathe her in, inhale some of the innocence in the hope it can cancel out my new harsh reality. My quilt has four special squares, one on each side, representing different parts of my 18-year old life. One is for my initials, a little chewed by moths, another for the comedy mask, representing theatre; the third square has a string of musical notes dancing over the fabric and the last one shows an image of the house I was leaving behind, reminding me of home.

I grew up in a family that had a mother and a father and four children, and somehow that is what I thought I had replicated. But a marriage is made up of a million micro-actions and barely-there responses; hard work and a little luck, tiny kindnesses that filter through the day like light through a blind. A marriage is not a thing you can cut and paste.

It is kindness I am craving now as I drive down the street towards the flat that will hold my children for the weekend, a horror film playing in my head. And I wonder, as I drive, how I am supposed to find my own story, woven as it is amongst those of my husband and my children. How can my story be excavated from the mine of my life when so much of it has been devoted to others? How can my truth find its way out of the tunnel and into the light, when I have lost myself in someone else?

Once home, the light has fallen behind the horizon, lost for another night. At the end of the street, beyond the allotments, a glowing sliver hangs in the air, like a smile. I throw my bag in through the front door and pull my coat around me. The night is crisp on my cheeks and coal smoke floats into the air. I walk down the street, where the sky is obscured by tree branches and something magical is taking place. It is impossible to discern any layers of cloud: everything is drenched in ink. But slowly a huge shadow is lifting and the Wolf Moon is emerging. Only one night after it reached its full power, the moon still appears whole, a perfect circle, and it is all the more mesmerising for the delay. Now I feel my heart hammering in my chest and my breath quickening. I look around for someone to share the moment with, but it is just me: a woman gazing at the Wolf Moon, still rising and completely free of the clouds.

2
Snow Moon

Storm Moon, Ice Moon

The sky is icy blue tonight, reflecting snow that has frozen hard on the ground as temperatures plummet. I have been lying in bed with my very darkest thoughts, and now walk to the landing barefoot, swallowing down demons. I open the window overlooking the back lane and gaze south. The air is illuminated with the promise of something wonderful just out of sight, too light to be midnight in February. But there is no crescent hanging sleepily above my house, only an illusion created by snow, beckoning a witching hour that has yet to begin. The true darkness is inside my head, and tonight there are no stars to pull me out of the abyss.

The crease between my ring finger and the palm of my hand is soft and tender against my thumbnail. I used to have a habit of absent-mindedly stroking my wedding ring as I stared at telegraph lines swaying against the sky, or leaned on the kitchen counter watching steam evaporate from the kettle. For a while there was still a groove in my finger where the ring had curled around it: my body still grieving for a loss that has proved harder to diffuse in my mind. The ring was yellow gold, slightly bevelled and scuffed. Bought in Hatton Gardens on a lunch break, just around the corner from the market stalls of Leather Lane, where fabrics and spices floated on the fume-filled breeze. Two giddy kids spending money they didn't have, pretending to be grown-ups.

I can still smell the sickly sweet cleaning fluids that ran in rivulets along the edge of the pavements and into the drains. Every morning, I would board the 38 bus from Hackney Central towards Dalston Junction, a kind of exotic wilderness full of chicken shops and newsagents. I knew never to walk alone here; it wasn't far from Murder Mile, a stretch of road permanently peppered with yellow crime signs.

The houses would grow steadily more gentrified as the bus meandered into Islington. Honey brickwork was carefully pointed and the front doors had brass knockers instead of a patchwork of doorbells at the side. There were parks too, blossom falling behind black railings and office workers pushing three-wheeled buggies. Mobile phones had become a thing, and I would play games on my Nokia 3310 as the bus crawled onto Essex Road. Low level flats and community gardens defined this road, the poor relation to Upper Street, which ran parallel, imbued with a golden New Labour haze. People jumped on and off the old Routemaster between stops, exhaust fumes curling around the metal pole at the back of the bus.

At Angel, the *Electrowerkz* nightclub lurked inside the old metal works building behind the tube station. At weekends my friends and I would blow the night apart with dance, drink and basslines at clubs like this one. Entering the room was like falling into an explosion; a whirling thrash of bodies surging around the bar, barely missing tables heaving with empty glasses. Heeled shoes and filthy, naked feet ground into the sticky floor, hands pumped the air. There were benefits to sleeping with the DJ, but now I look back, when I thought I was owning the dancefloor, really I was dancing in his shadow.

Next the bus would nudge over a heaving crossroads, turning past Sadlers Wells, where I would ring the bell and trip down the stairs, alighting at Mount Pleasant post office. From there, it was only a couple of minutes to the white office full of Japanese art and Converse trainers.

Occasionally on a lunchtime I would take a walk. Not for long, because I didn't get paid if I wasn't at my desk and I needed the hours on my timesheet. But long enough to watch the butchers staggering out of *The Hope* opposite Smithfield Market, aprons smudged with blood, hands as raw as the meat they sold. Long enough to wander up to Leather Lane and trail my fingers through racks of harem pants and layered skirts. And long enough to continue along Hatton Gardens, where I would choose the plainest gold band in the shop.

The act of removing the ring turned out to be just as painful as our final embrace. My finger was red and swollen, like my daughters eyes, and I can still feel the metal squeezing my knuckle as it slid slowly off, soap bubbles reflecting rainbows. I thought I had forgotten what it is to wear a wedding ring, how much of a statement it is of belonging. There was security in it for a time, but in the end it became a visceral, gaudy reminder of everything that had gone wrong.

The ring now lies in an egg-shaped box, underneath a lock of my youngest daughter's baby hair. When I hold it I can see that it is beautiful: delicate and simple. I stroke the space where that ring once lived, and it is sad, but somehow the absence feels kinder.

The air is growing warmer. No longer an icy blast as I open the door to release the cat each morning. I stand for a moment, leaning on the door frame, and try to sense the mood of the day. There seems to be less security in the lightening sky: I am no longer protected by the pinprick light of endless stars, and the days are rushing in quick and hard.

At night I hear a tap tap tap on the wall next to my head. Sometimes I am asleep and the sound will crawl around my dream until I jolt awake with a little gasp. Swinging my feet onto cool floorboards, I stumble into my older daughters' bedroom, where The Mermaid lies pinned to her sheets, eyes darting, breath shallow. Her legs have stopped working, attacked by a virus we were told doesn't affect children, but also perhaps a manifestation of the fear inhabiting her mind. We lie in the dark together, a mother holding her little girl tight, squeezing away the ghosts, willing them to flee on the breath of a tumble of lullabies. Slowly, her breathing becomes deeper, her muscles relax and I slip from her bed and tiptoe away, hoping for a few hours of sleep before it all starts again.

The whole household is developing a hypervigilance that echoes that of my poorly daughter, constantly watching and checking to make sure she is safe. Her eyes can glaze over in a heartbeat as she disappears into a world that terrifies her, one where she can never be safe. And I will quickly step in to pull her back before she falls too far, though often it is too late, and she has gone. And then the shaking will start, and the rocking, and a concerned little sister will bring a teddy for her to hold, as if squeezing it would fix everything. If only. And another sister will ask *is she ok?* And I will say *she's fine, why don't you see if you can find a game to play? Don't worry your sister is fine*. And The Whirlwind, the one with the brain like lightning, knows that it's all starting again and her sister is not ok at all, and her cheeks start to flush and she will do anything to make it stop. Anything to make her sister come back from the underworld.

Much of my time as a mother has been spent trying to explain why my eldest daughter can not fit into the place determined for her by society. The Mermaid started school when she was four and I deregistered her when she was six. Those two years ultimately created such a sense of trauma and mistrust around formal education that I have never managed to find a school placement where she can thrive.

I would stand in the playground while she lined up, a tiny dot of a girl in a dark pink coat with tears dripping into the fur-lined hood. She didn't just sob, she screamed for me, eyes wide with terror, while the teacher shushed her and led her away. At playtimes she scoured the playground for sycamore seeds, meticulously picking them up and storing them in her pockets. Each evening when I looked inside her book bag, helicopters would pour onto the kitchen table, falling on the wood or scattering across the floor as if they were desperate to escape.

The Mermaid grew pale. Her tummy ached and she woke with nightmares still racing through her head. I had never had a school-age child before but I didn't think this was what she was supposed to look like, a shadow-girl shrinking before my eyes. The head teacher told me I was making her anxious with my own concerns, which became a theme that grew into a monster. I have been told repeatedly by health and education professionals that I make my child anxious, some kind of Munchausen-by-proxy intimation designed to induce fear and confusion. A special type of gaslighting that conveniently conceals the reality.

In the classroom, The Mermaid was teaching her peers to read because she had already whipped through every book on the shelf. *She's working way beyond expectation* they told me, as if that made everything ok. Years later I am still arguing that outstanding intelligence is of very little use when a child's spirit is crushed.

It would be several more years before I started to realise that her brain digested life differently to me, in a way
I was desperate to understand. The challenges she faced
were underpinned by autism, hidden behind a mask at a
huge cost to her health.

When I deregistered her from school it was in order to
save her, to find the daughter who had got lost inside the
school system, but it was also with a sense of optimism
that education could be something better. I was persuaded
by literature I read about child-led learning and unschool-
ing. Ken Robinson's TedTalk about the importance of
finding a passion in life rang in my ears. I had two other
tiny daughters who could learn alongside her and a
husband who seemed to be along for the ride. We would
be a tribe, and we would make The Mermaid's unhappi-
ness a catalyst for positive change, a better way of doing
things.

For a time there was so much to love about home
education. I spent days pounding the sands with a tiny
Caulbearer strapped to my chest, a Whirlwind splashing
along the shoreline and a Mermaid searching for herself
in the reflection of endless pieces of sea glass. Our learning became an extension of my mothering, forcing me to
see life through their eyes and question everything I had
learned about education during my own teacher-training.
Kitchen walls were strewn with displays, numbers painted
on doorways, mobiles dangling from the ceiling, models
precariously balanced on top of the piano. Trips to
Culloden battlefield and random prehistorical sites I had

discovered online late at night. Taking the train to the city to attend an art group, breastfeeding in a museum while small daughters lay on tummies and gazed up at Egyptian Mummies.

We were almost invincible, our tribe, and I became used to deflecting questions about our family, and why we looked a little different. It's funny how ignorance can sometimes look a lot like fear. At the time I thought strangers' enquiring eyes were mirroring my own uncertainty, but now I understand it was me they were frightened of, my questioning of everything they thought they knew. I was strong, with fire in my eyes, I just didn't know it.

The flip side of living The Good Life is that it can be very easy to lose yourself. That is probably true of many parents of small children destroyed by milk-soaked nights, but, for us, the complete immersion in family life required by home education magnified the challenges. My relationship was already slipping away from me at this point. A crack was appearing between my expectations of marriage and children and the reality. I thought we were a team, committed to raising children together and supporting each other in creative work endeavours, but I seemed to have fallen into a gender trap. For all the liberal chatter over glasses of red wine and niche vinyl, our roles had become wholly conventional and I resented that hugely. It was becoming clear that my dreams were exactly that, *my* dreams, not ours. So when another baby was thrown into the mix, things only got messier.

*   *   *

For a time, I lose the moon, it has been stolen by the clouds. But one night I open my front door and tiptoe round the corner of my street, and there it is, hanging deft and cheeky like a smirk. And I am confused. This Snow Moon seems elusive, difficult to place. It could be, I reason illogically, that the moon itself is muddled. The snow has, after all, melted. Temperatures are rising rapidly and may well be causing some kind of lunar identity crisis. As the planet burns, snow is no longer guaranteed and seems, in recent years, to fall later in the year.

But as the month drags on, in a fester of psychological drama and domestic turmoil, the night sky becomes more familiar. As the full moon approaches, I am once more able to sit at my desk, where spider plants fall, and look up at the circular glow, with its familiar face shining down on my tired heart. If I stare through my window for long enough, a smaller reflection of the moon appears, and I imagine we are communicating, as if I am inhabiting its reflection and the sky between us is only a heartbeat. If I move my head, the reflection bobs around as I control it with my stare. My wide eyes beckon the moon closer, until an oystercatcher flies over the lane, chattering noisily and breaking the spell.

A couple of days earlier, I had managed to escape the house and grind my feet into sandy cliff tops. Running past the static caravans, I tripped through the grass onto the beach. It was low tide and the sand was sprawled with sandpipers and oystercatchers pecking for food, beaks submerged then victorious. The air was mild but blustery, the type of wind that comes at you sideways and blows right inside your ear. I felt a frustration brewing, caused by listless children, half-finished ideas and grey sky, and the beach was swept with endless brown seaweed, which didn't help. Two cuddy ducks rose up from the rock pools, and I almost collided with a skitter of sanderlings as I ran hard along the shoreline. I am normally quick to cry, but today everything was buried deep and dark inside until I ran up off the beach and paused by the curlew field. Today it seemed bare, a waterlogged scrub, when I noticed movement just beyond the fence. A huge jack hare, ears smudged black, turned towards me and everything shifted. Unsure if my cheeks were wet from drizzle or tears, I breathed and breathed and smiled at last and everything was lighter. We watched each other, the hare and I, then ran our separate ways.

In an attempt to extinguish the ghosts that continue to haunt me, I try, a little reluctantly, to engage with a new therapist. I want to locate my whisper amongst the shouts drowning me out. My truth tends to float away from me just when I need it most, like waves carrying me further from the shore when I swim. The current knocks me off course, breeze blowing ripples sideways, and I find myself in a different place from the one I imagined.

There can be no face to face contact, so I feed my children and send them upstairs to put on their pyjamas and pull down the blinds. I cut up apples, fill beakers with milk and find a film that the little girls will love and the older ones will watch without too much resentment. And I am proud when the daughter who pounds her feet for the moon fusses around her sisters and tells them that this is Mummy's special time and they must *sit quietly and give her some space*. This daughter understands the value of caring for oneself. Or perhaps she is keen to ensure that her mother retains a semblance of sanity, and knows full well the necessity of fifty minutes of venting. Whatever, the scene is set for an opportunity for me to find myself and feel validated, and I light a candle and push the door against the world.

The therapist is Greek, with a strong accent wrapping her words like a gift. I am surprised that the atmosphere between me and my laptop is charged, so that after I have cried, gut-wrenching sobs that burst from my soul, the silence is precious and meaningful. We breathe together, the therapist and I, and it feels like a caress, a kindness that has been missing. And then my children pile into the room, pink-cheeked and bickering, and I hold them all close, long blonde hair in my mouth and elbows in my ribs, and it is everything. They are everything.

This month, I am mainly confined to my home, fiercely guarding The Mermaid like a tiger, but also caged and frustrated as I breath the same air again and again. Across the country, eyes meet through screens and people are becoming accustomed to absences that feel like a constant ache in the stomach or a flutter in the chest. There is a solidarity to this crisis that is laced with desperation, as we sit tight and wait for the horror to dissipate.

The monotonous laps of the back lane feel too risky while The Mermaid is so ill. I can turn my back for a minute and my smallest daughter will run down the stairs, *Mummy come quickly*! And my heartbeat quickens as frightened whimpers, muted by the duvet, squeak from a curled up ball on the bed. And I tell The Littlest One *it's fine, she's ok, don't worry*, but The Mermaid emerges and stares at me with wide watery eyes and flushed cheeks because it's not fine at all.

On the weekend of the Snow Moon, the three youngest daughters are with their father, and The Mermaid and I drive 60 miles south-west into County Durham, across miles of moorland to visit my parents. The brazen starkness of these northernmost counties has started to feel something like home. There's an air of wild abandon in these vast, barren stretches of land. When I drive into Weardale, the world opens out below me, like I could fall off the edge. And beyond Stanhope, where my parents' house sits tilted on a steep hill, the road meanders along a plateau almost 2000m above sea level, slowly winding down across cattle grids into a valley. The girls call this part of the drive the middle of nowhere - *are we in the middle of nowhere yet Mummy*?

I still question our move from London to the wild north-east, fuelled by a lack of money and mice scratching inside in the walls. We were broke and the van we hired wasn't big enough. One of my brothers would later end up accompanying my husband back down the M1 to pick up a second load, fuelled by Detroit techno and KFC.

It was dark when I strapped the baby in next to me in the front of the van. The red lights at the top of Telecom Tower taunted me beyond the car park, flirting and daring me to escape from its seductive flash. A train rumbled past, light from the windows framing weary faces returning from night shifts, heads leaning on reinforced glass, eyes closed. Our flat would shake whenever a train went past: vibrations could be felt through the floor that we could never afford to carpet. On the other side of the track lived a family of foxes. I enjoyed watching the three cubs roll down the bank while their mother looked on. We became mothers together.

I didn't feel sad when I locked the door for the last time, although my baby had been born in that flat, her slippery body bursting out of me into the water. And I didn't feel sad when we drove out of the gates, past the fishmongers and the bakery with its synthetic cream cakes. I didn't even feel sad when we left Nunhead Library behind, where I had wheeled my daughter in her buggy most days, willing her to sleep for just twenty minutes so I could log on to my emails and reconnect with the person I was before I was a mother.

It wasn't until a couple of days later that I realised what I had left behind, and the swirling in my stomach spread as a cold chill up to my shoulders. I wonder now if this was the moment when everything changed. We both felt it, my husband and I, an uncomfortable dread, as we trudged through claggy mud up a disused railway line in County Durham. Here was the fresh air we had been dreaming of, but the grass wasn't greener. It was scuffed with dirt, and stubborn clouds hung close to the ground, hiding the sunshine we had imagined. This was the moment when I should have realised that change can only come from within, that a new house won't quell that restlessness, however pretty the garden. Itchy feet, he used to call it, my inability to stay still and inhabit the present. I could never be mindful but I still had so much to learn. I was a child inhabiting a woman's body and playing house. Overthinking was my sport, but I had not actually stopped to consider my choices in life, or the impact of moving out of the city. I felt like a fraud, a fish out of water, drowning in air.

We arrive at my parents' in time for me to throw on running gear and settle The Mermaid on a sofa. One of the many intrigues of my daughter's brain is the speed at which it moves. This is an advantage when it comes to playing Scrabble with her grandfather, or devouring books, but the downside is that it travels so fast it rarely slows down: the momentum is so huge that the information hurtles around like a cat chasing its tail. Her memory is photographic: she can recite text she has seen only once or twice and retain complex information very easily. But she is also the elephant who never forgets, and her exhausted brain holds and distorts feelings and historical exchanges until they loom like monsters and take on lives of their own. It is these demons that haunt her, and the combination of a lightning brain and a blocked filter is causing endless pain.

Tonight, however, she focuses on the dictionary inside her head. With a determination to win Scrabble and a huge love for my father, The Mermaid will curl up on a cushion like a cat and feel safe with her grandad while my mother and I hunt down the Snow Moon.

People say I look like my mum, but I don't see myself when I look into her eyes. Like the many strands that make up a marriage and determine whether or not it will last the distance, my unique genetic combination means that any similarities I have to my mum have been woven around my own identity. It would be lazy to describe her as the strong, calm force that underpins our family, though she is that. But just as every woman in history is more than a building block for other people's success, my mum has a story of her own. As a child her lack of confidence was more visible than mine, but that probably suggests an awareness missing from my own character. While my uncertainties buried themselves beneath layers of drama and smiles, my mother slowly grew into herself. It would have been easy for her to be lost in the shadows cast by my dad's bright light but she just kept burning harder. Maybe I hoped that marriage meant being ignited by someone else's flame, but now I can see that I was already flickering hard, only to be snuffed out.

*   *   *

Despite the rise in temperatures across the country, seams of snow puncture the landscape where it has fallen so deep and hard it won't shift in a hurry. There is some cloud cover, and I have been glancing up at the sky all day, wondering whether the Snow Moon will be visible tonight.

As my mum and I drive to the top of the middle of nowhere, smoke rises from the moor: heather is being burned. Flames lick the ground and clouds of white smoke float in front of my eyes. The burning fills my nostrils, even from inside the car. Mum parks outside a remote café where a family sits at a picnic table and a man is stroking his dog's ears. From this spot, high up in the dale, we can see the sky turning blush red beyond the North Pennines in the west. The valley stretches for miles, slashed by stubborn snow. It's hard not to stand and gaze at the flaming hills, but the Snow Moon will not rise from the west, we must run the other way with the sunset flashing at our heels.

We leave the café and the family and the dog behind, tasting the smoke, which is filling the sky all round us now as we run. Over to the east, the lights of old industrial powerhouses are starting to flicker; Consett is a telephone switchboard, and an aerial glows red like a traffic light. There are wind turbines too, but the air is almost completely still, so they don't spin and the smoke won't shift. On a clear day, you can see right across to the coast, to Sunderland where the River Wear pours itself into the North Sea, and to Newcastle and Gateshead, divided by the mighty Tyne. Not tonight though. I must content myself with the burning sky behind me, and as I run I crane my neck and inhale the explosion of colour.

The track we are running on is stone-dashed and fairly flat, and the moor rolls down on one side to a reservoir. There is no one else around, just the odd car in the distance and some grouse belching in the heather. As we reach a slight incline, the path is piled high with snow, still white and hard, but bathed in a rosy glow.

At the crest of the hill, there is no sign of the moon. A faint tinge of burning singes the air, but it's fresh up here. We are running towards a copse of trees. It is shadowy against the lights of the town because the sky is darkening now. Behind us, the sunset has deepened and is starting to bleed into the night. It is almost time to turn back.

And then I scream. *Look*! I shout to my mother. *It's there!*

And we stand together, gasping the last air of the day. Beyond the patchwork of lights, a gauzy orb is shimmering through the mist. It is barely there, reflecting the sunset on its surface, which is glowing iridescent pink. Rising oh so slowly, the Snow Moon is majestic and confident - even a million fires burning on these moors couldn't smother her. Sweat is cooling on our bodies as a flock of curlews pecks around in a field, barely visible in the fading light.

The bag of Scrabble tiles will be empty. Reluctantly, we must turn our backs on the moon and return. And as we run, we chat. Sometimes I sprint ahead in bursts of energy then circle back to meet my mother, taking another opportunity to watch the Snow Moon as it rises higher, craters and valleys visible like veins. And then, for a time, the moon is enveloped in indigo cloud, and we run on in darkness, head torches bobbing beams of light onto the snowy path.

The reservoir lies ahead. Above us the sky is inky vastness and stars are pricking the darkness. We stand and breathe, tired now, the chilly air grabbing at our bones. As we look back, the Snow Moon is emerging from the clouds, no longer dipped pink, but glowing ivory, edges blurring if we stare too long. A curlew overhead might witness some kind of dance, as we stare and whoop and raise our eyes to the stars.

3
Lenten Moon

Plough Moon, Wind Moon, Death Moon,
Chaste Moon, Lengthening Moon

I am sleeping. The house is silent. Not even the sound of the cat's soft, lapping tongue stealing my water as I fall into a dream. A log cabin backs onto pine trees and opens up at the front onto a yellowish field leading to some kind of mansion. Mountains, like the ones I saw in a children's picture book the other day, jut purple and hard against the smudged sky. I am on a holiday, the kind I talk about all the time, a remote cottage in Scotland. My children are with me, and my oldest daughter is running around on her mermaid legs. So it must be a dream.

There is a knock at the door. A blurred figure can be seen through the frosted glass, smiling at me as fresh air smacks my face. She is holding a strange contraption that locks and unlocks not only the front door but also my car. How helpful! The visitor must be the lady of the manor, she is all confidence and riding boots and not used to people questioning her. *You must come out for tea*, says the lady of the manor. *Bring the girls - four daughters, imagine! - and I'll show you the local pub, come on!* And somehow, without realising it, we are walking up to a pub and the lady's husband and several children and dogs have appeared.

The pub is tatty, with a weird menu. I help my children choose drinks that include pieces of cut up fruit. Despite it being a dream, my tiny third daughter, The Caulbearer, is indecisive and takes forever to choose from the menu, and this makes it feel more realistic. The girls run off to play and revel in the holiday newness of it all while I chat with the woman and her husband. The husband is relaxed and friendly, and it is enjoyable when he walks behind where I am sitting and softly kisses my neck. Enjoyable but shocking, because the wife is looking at me as if this might be fine, challenging me with her eyes. And, loving the sensation of his lips upon my skin, I feel desired and secure, because I know it is a dream, and the children are all well and happy. And I wonder if I feel safe because the lady is offering to gift her husband, who seems kind and decent? The lady is saying *you deserve this, allow yourself to be desired just for a few hours, accept him as a delightful interlude.* And then she disappears. *You won't see us again.*

On the night of the new moon, when the Lenten Moon is sandwiched between the Earth and the Sun, the sky is clear. Across the country, candles in jars are being placed on doorsteps and windowsills. A man, a police officer, has snatched a woman from the street as she walked home, and he has killed her. The woman's body has been found in a builder's bag in woodland, which is unimaginable, and her smiling face shines out of newspapers.

Women are angry and women are scared, and women want to be together in solidarity, to feel each other's strength and warmth. But the police say no.

NO.

You may not gather at a safe social distance and remember this woman, you may not express your grief, you must stay behind closed doors where you belong. We don't want to see your wild eyes and fierce jaws. If you try to gather we will brutalise you and whip you up into a frenzy, just to remind the world that women become hysterical and shrill when they are upset. It is best if you stay inside. Keep yourselves safe. Protect yourselves. And so the insistence of the passive continues, placing the onus on women to be proactive in preventing the violent actions of men.

I have no idea how to explain any of this to my daughters. I don't want to scare them. There will be time enough for that when they begin to walk out on their own, hearts bumping in chests, blood rushing through ears, feet quickening at the sound of cars. That fear will be a backdrop to their lives, no need to expedite it. But The Mermaid already understands, and she makes a banner for Sarah Everard, paints it black, and places it in the living room window.

At 9.30pm that night, I light a candle and place it carefully on the wall outside my home, hoping the breeze will allow the flames to flicker for a while in this nationwide vigil. The street is empty. Perhaps everyone else feels safe. I breathe and look up at the stars, imagining candles burning up and down the country, their glow reflected in tear-filled eyes. The silence in my tiny front garden is deafening, and I want to run down the street banging on doors and demanding to know why every one of them is not burning candles and howling in anger. But behind the curtains, televisions are flickering and dogs curl on rugs. Maybe a woman walks on eggshells, or strokes a bruised arm, but no one can see. No one knows. Just like no one knows about the times I wake suddenly in the middle of the night with a lump in my chest and a bird in my throat. Roughly dragged from my always-light sleep by voices outside my window or a car engine running nearby. The fear doesn't come from nowhere, it trickles through lives because there is good reason to be scared.

The next Monday evening, the two youngest girls are bouncing around on my bed. There are teddies, bedtime stories and hot water bottles. Children skip in and out of the room, make faces in the mirror and carry the cat around, who tries not to protest. The Littlest One hides a tooth under a pillow for fairies to whisk away in the moonlight. The Caulbearer stands thoughtfully under a framed lunar calendar that hangs on the wall. She is checking the carefully painted orbs and crescents to see what sort of moons our birthdays will bring.

Caul bearers are rare nowadays. Modern births involve more intervention, and the membranes are often broken before the baby emerges. This one was born in a pool on a stone floor, surprising the midwife with her speedy arrival. *It's not time yet* she said, as I reached down to feel the head between my legs. My fingers stroked a soft, fleshy bulge, nothing like a head at all. No time to be alarmed though because another contraction coursed through my body, and my baby girl emerged, translucent membranes covering her from head to toe. The midwife used some kind of hook to break the caul and reveal the face, and my baby screamed fierce cries as the onslaught of cooler air wrapped around her body.

The little girl stands there now in her spotted nightie, eyes raised to the moons on the wall. I saved the caul and placed it carefully between sheets of baking paper. It is packed in a box in the loft, because I know that a caul is precious, often carried by sailors on ships as a talisman against drowning. But whilst it is an enviable gift, in the past being born with the 'veil of tears' led to persecution; these precious babes were believed to be witches or heretics and treated with ignorance and violence. Men were scared of something they didn't understand.

This caul bearer is a mysterious child who experiences life deeply. Quiet and thoughtful, hilarious and stubborn, perhaps she knows something others don't. On the beach, she will run to the very edge of the shore and stand on a rock as the waves splash at her legs. Her white blonde hair will blow around her face and she will look out to sea as the breeze catches her sleeves. She will stay there for some time, while her sisters play pirates or splash in rock pools. And when she returns to me her cheeks will be rosy and her eyes will hold a gleam, as if she has been replenished.

The next day starts the same as any other. We are on the other side of yet another lockdown and I set an alarm so that I rise an hour before the children must be woken for school. I use my middle finger to wipe the grit from the corner of my eye, clearing the way for a new day. I feel slightly nauseous from lack of sleep, but this hour is precious, the only time when no one needs me.

I feel a soft weight on the edge of the bed, and the cat pads up to me, nudging my face with a wet nose and whiskers. I lie there, bones sinking deep into the mattress, weighed down by a thousand thoughts, then force myself to push the duvet away and reach for my glasses. Tying my hair into a bun on the top of my head, I pour myself into my dressing gown. The floorboards are cool under my feet and they creak as I head downstairs.

Every morning when the the stairs creak I remember the times I crept down to the lounge in the middle of the night, in the days before I slept in the smallest room in the house. I would wake in the early hours and the other side of the double bed would be empty and cold. My mind would quicken as my body flooded with a visceral mixture of sadness, anxiety and disappointment that this was my life. Tiptoeing downstairs, the carpet runner rough against my feet, I would lean my body into the wall, try to push my weight away from the stairs to stop the creaking.

Some nights he would jump as I entered the room. He would have headphones on and be crouching over a laptop, always the laptop reflecting his eyes when I wanted him to be staring into my own. Every time the stairs creak, I wonder if I should call someone to come and fix them, bang nails into the wood until the squeaking stops. Keep hammering until I can't hear it anymore.

My counsellor has told me to write down three things each day that I appreciate, and already this feels like another job I must add to my extremely long list. It is in my nature to flit between thoughts, and I can find it hard to focus on one thing at a time. But I want to do better, to be better, so I add it mentally to my list of things to do.

In one counselling session, I arrive at the screen looking hollow and ancient, skin grey with wounded holes for eyes. The older children are watching telly downstairs, the little girls are playing princesses just across the hall with a book that folds out into a palace.

I have pushed my bedroom door closed. The door is broken so sometimes it pops open and a burst of cool air will enter the room, usually followed by a small child clutching a teddy. This evening though I am crying so hard, trying not to make a noise, that I desperately hope the door will stay shut and the fold-out book will work its magic.

I am crying because I am scared, and I can't work out how not to be scared. Word-sobs fall from my mouth and crawl under the bed to fester amongst the dust and discarded hair bobbles. It's possible that the fear has always been there, manifesting itself as vicious nightmares all through my childhood. It comes from a place I have inhabited for so long it feels like a toxic friendship I can't quite shake, years of trying to make myself heard. And now I spend my days being challenged by professionals and trying to rebuild a fractured life, and the result is a woman who has lost faith in those childish notions that life is fair, or that doing your best is enough. Because it has not been enough to save me or my children and so maybe my best is not my best at all, because everything is so broken. And this is why I am crying. I am so full of loathing for my own weakness that the counsellor's face seems to have taken on a mask of impatience, and I understand again what it means to cry as if your heart will break.

At last the sobbing stops and I am left with skin that is reddened and puffy, my breath ragged and sore. The counsellor's mask has dropped, and she now looks gently concerned through the pixels on the screen. No one speaks. Slowly my shoulders fall and the counsellor asks me what I notice. *I feel empty now* I say, *there is nothing left.* And it feels good to have got those demons out, although they are only floating around the room, they have not left completely. *Remember that emptiness, that space,* says the counsellor, just as the broken door pops open and two little girls run in.

* * *

The lunar calendar tells me that the Lenten Moon should be emerging, waxing crescent. The term Lenten is clearly linked to the Christian calendar, that barren time after the pancakes have all been eaten, lemon squeezed and sugar licked from the plate. But it derives originally from the Old English word, *lencten*, for spring. Quite literally it means the lengthening of the days as the sun's light lingers in the sky, and I am trying hard to feel the benefit and not crawl back into the darkness.

Christianity used to punctuate my week as a child, with church choir practice on a Friday evening and at least one service on a Sunday, sometimes a wedding on a Saturday when I would sit in the choir stalls and marvel at the lace and the gauze wrapped around the bride. I loved the choir, the ritual of the ruff around the neck and the starched white surplice. The burgundy cassocks that held the sweat and dust of previous inhabitants, and pinched under the arms. I learned a lot from Mr Crinall, hunched and cantankerous, and wispy Mr Lambie, the choir masters who taught us psalms, anthems and descants in the freezing vestry. I had girlish crushes on boy choristers and blushed when they looked at me across the aisle. And the whole ceremony of it appealed to my sense of melodrama, offering me a chance to perform and the space to dream. Ave Marias floating up into the chancel and candles burning. Always candles.

It seems ridiculous to me now, the parading around the aisles, following a brass cross held high on a wooden pole. But religion stayed with me until just after my wedding. I clung to it because it had meant something to my wider family, through death and illness, but now all that remains is the music, the voices and the rules of the harmonies. The notes were mainly crafted by men, and that bothers me now. Where were the soft soprano voices soaring and dropping like skylarks? Were they confined to lullabies sung at the crib, while deep alto tones floated into fireplaces as fingers knitted rows? Or were they strangled out by the purity of childish treble tones, the presence of women in the choir stalls too shocking to consider? Where are these women's voices, the stories they told? Despite this, Stanford and Steiner, Purcell and Parry used to be part of me, and they took me to a place where I was completely vulnerable, laid bare behind the altar as I watched the breaking of the body of Christ, the drinking of his blood. Such strange rituals, drenched in patriarchy, inspiring fear and awe, but there was something about the darkness even then that held me tight. Also the history. I would stroke the polished wood that held my books, notice the symmetry of the carvings, the dust that settled in crevices and the scent of polish that floated in the air. The church organ still alternately intrigues and oppresses me.

My mother sends a photo of the Lenten Moon curling in a cornflower blue sky. I have not yet seen this one, it must be hiding on the other side of the house beyond the end of the terrace. Evenings are full of children and zooms and there is no time for moons.

* * *

After school, with the weather getting warmer, the allotment beckons. I have always dreamed of my own garden,
of a back door that opens onto grass and holds my children safe. When my daughters were tiny I trawled through
Rightmove looking for the perfect house with a lawn at
the back, but it didn't exist within our budget. And
anyway, even the perfect house couldn't mend a marriage.

Since I have been on my own I have had a fence built
around my postage stamp front garden. I painted it sage
green and planted lavender and roses in the border. In the
summer I throw down blankets and the children cover
them with Sylvanian Families and books, while I bring
out bowls of pasta and cups of water that spill onto the
grass. The neighbours over the road call this 'the dark side
of the street', because the sun doesn't hit these houses
until later on in the afternoon. In the winter my miniature
garden barely sees the sun at all. But during the precious
summer months this side of the street is perfect for lazy
evenings and a glass of wine on the bench. If it's a beautiful morning, I will take my coffee onto the lane at the
back of the house, perch on the step next to the bins and
stretch my legs out on the tarmac. Sometimes the girls
will chalk patterns on the lane or lie on rugs and draw.
They are like cats, chasing the warmth, there's always a
patch of sunlight if they look hard enough.

* * *

At night, the cat occasionally stays out wandering. There is no cat flap, so someone must open the door to let her in or out. Sometimes she sits at the lounge window, eyes intense and staring, ivy brushing her spotted fur. Other times, one of my daughters will open the front door and call her name, and she will dart out from under the car with a mew and trot through their legs.

At bedtime, if the cat is not home, I pull on my long woollen coat over my dressing gown, push my feet into whichever shoes are lying next to the front door and step into the night. I carefully lock the door behind me, even though I am only walking to the end of my road and I keep looking over my shoulder, check that I can still see my house containing all of my children behind the blinds. Just a minute on my own to shed my skin.

On this particular night, the street is quiet. A few windows leak light through curtains. A car passes along the main road, tyres brushing the tarmac. I look up at the sky, encouraging my eyes to ignore the glare from the street-lamps. It has been a pleasant early spring day, and tonight there are no clouds, just a sea of stars bobbing in the black. I turn towards the west, and there it is, in its first quarter: Lenten Moon.

My shoulders drop a little. It has been another day of meetings with a psychiatrist and a very poorly daughter, back in the room with chipped cream walls and the moss green chair where the psychiatrist sat behind his laptop. Behind a mask, sitting tense in her wheelchair, my daughter's eyes were either hollow or desperate, maybe

47

both, I couldn't tell. She had written her horror in tiny words onto a page torn from a glittery notebook. This is how she lets the psychiatrist know that fitting into this world feels too hard, the drugs are not working. I interrogated the psychiatrist and I advocated for my daughter and I pushed her through the town in her wheelchair to collect the new, stronger prescription of drugs. And I swallowed my fire down when the chemist asked me if I knew what a strong dose this was that I was requesting for my young daughter, because of course I knew, and of course I didn't want to be asking for it. I wanted to be watching my daughter treading carefully around the barnacles, long hair stroking her waist as she lowered herself into the rockpool and laughed at the cold. This was not the plan.

It is this sadness I am exhaling into the night as I turn away from the moon and my house and walk to the far end of the street, where a patchwork of allotments lies in a strip above the supermarket. Sometimes the clanging of lorries unpacking deliveries can be heard and it upsets the people living at this end of the street, but tonight there is no noise except for my feet crunching over stones as I walk along the lane. I whistle and call, waiting for two circles of light to flash on the fence, or a telltale rustle in the bushes. Nothing. I walk a little further along the lane, which is unlit. I remember a few months ago a woman was assaulted just around the corner on the bridge and my babysitter texted me to tell me to be careful. I am not being careful tonight, I don't see why I should. I have read somewhere that there is a Hunger Moon, and tonight it feels like every moon in the sky is a Hunger Moon. Some men don't ever seem to lose their appetite. It feels like the anger of a million women is simmering under my skin and if anyone grabbed me now I would destroy them with fingernails of fire as my wild hair tied them in knots. Despite this, instinct tells me to glance over my shoulder and I am relieved when a tiny shadow bounds towards me and it is my cat.

We play a game, the cat and I, as we walk back towards the house: I follow the pavement in a straight line while the cat darts in and out of the cars, running ahead to wait and then bounding back. I look up at the sky one more time. As I stare, the moon becomes a star, light bleeding out, reaching towards me. I unlock my door and step inside.

In the year when the world became smaller, and adventures had to be found closer to home, I became a little addicted to swimming in wild water. I discovered that icy dips helped The Mermaid to regulate, and the sight of her at ease and fearless fuelled my addiction. I scoured maps for pools in the hills and led my tribe of daughters through forests in search of hidden waterfalls. I found a rockpool surrounded by barnacles and oystercatchers that was a secret infinity pool: at the right angle, swimming towards the sea, I felt like I could swim right off the edge of the earth, beyond the tilt where the water meets the sky. Other times, when the clouds were heavy and the tide a little higher, waves would crash over the rocks into the pool and delight me, splashing into my face and rocking me backwards and forwards. It was in this pool that The Caulbearer bobbed with one orange armband, not quite trusting herself to manage without it, while The Littlest One clung like a limpet to my neck.

I have a photo, taken by The Whirlwind standing high above the rockpool, and in the photo I am laughing, clutching a little girl in a wetsuit. My oldest daughter is once more a mermaid, circling The Caulbearer, who bobs with her one armband. This picture represents some of my very best mothering. Behind the camera, there is a bag containing a thermos of hot chocolate, plastic cups and grapes, and soon I will wrap my shivering girls in towels and hold them tightly as they sip their drinks, feeling wild and proud.

I love this photo because I look brave, and I am showing my children how to be brave. I am completely inside the moment, not pulled in a thousand directions feeling like everything I do is barely adequate, and the moment is golden. The children and I still talk about that day in the rockpool, take the memory out and examine it when we need to.

Almost a year later, I drive my two youngest girls to school, tip them through the door with a kiss on each head and head down to the beach. My body is bone tired but I pound my feet to the top of the sand dunes, paying particular attention to the yellow gorse flowers and beach huts. Running back along the beach I spot a dead seal. Its teeth are bared, surprisingly long. Wiry whiskers protrude from the snout. The seal is high up the beach, beyond the shoreline, stomach matted with sand. A hole punctures the skin. I run on, leaving the seal behind, though it stays in my head for days afterwards.

Back at the car, I sit and wait for a friend, watching in the mirror for a red car that soon appears, winding down the lane from the village. This friend is a dancer. Her hair hangs long down a very straight back, and she is always graceful when she moves, even on the school run. Today the dancer and I are going to swim in the sea, the first time I have done so this year. I like to swim in only a costume, but my body isn't yet acclimatised to the low water temperature so we walk onto the beach and squeeze into shortie wetsuits, holding hair on heads and zipping each other up.

Someone walks past with a dog, but otherwise the beach is empty. Dunstanburgh Castle lies in shadow across the bay and the sun is starting to strain through the clouds, sending a silver thread across the water. I leap off a ledge of sand and run down to the sea. The water is so cold it burns my feet, actually hurts the nerves, stinging and pulsing against my skin. But the sea is clear and waves are breaking around our waists and the only thing to do is push forward as lungs turn to ice.

We are laughing and squealing now, trying to slow our breath, which is coming in gasps. As we swim away from the land the waves are a little bigger, and we ride them like rollercoasters, spinning in the surf. We are sea witches frolicking, spinning spells of salt and shells, washing away the everyday and reclaiming the magic.

That night, the Lenten Moon hangs high above the house, blurred by clouds that are blown quickly across the sky by a strengthening wind. The stars are buried, burning hard but not for me. The moon is still glowing though, reflecting the longing in my eyes. The cat is playing outside again, arching her back and leaping across the wall. Eventually I tempt her in with biscuits, and close the door on the night.

The school holidays are nearing and I take the younger three children to visit their father for a few days. When my car pulls up outside his flat in a trendy part of the city, where people drink coffee on pavements and a Waitrose sits on the corner, the girls jump out of the car clutching teddies and hide out of sight after knocking. They shriek when their father opens the door and he gasps in mock surprise. Meanwhile The Mermaid has curled herself into a tiny ball, made herself as small as she can, coiled up like the pearly snail shells that scatter the dunes. I unload a suitcase and a bag of wellies, and wrap my children around me, feeling their warm arms on my skin, inhaling their necks and white blonde fairy hair. I close my eyes tight and try to magic The Mermaid through the door with her sisters, make my life a little easier, make one less thing my fault. But all the spells in the world do not work and when I open my eyes she is still inside the car.

Every time I leave my daughters I remember that I stayed for so long because this was the thing I feared the most, not being with them. And the sense of freedom that I presumed must be the payoff, well that has never arrived, because the second the girls are through the door I return to the car and place my hands on the shaking legs of The Mermaid. Tell her that she is safe, ask her to put on her seat belt, turn on the radio and talk about what we will eat for tea that night. Sometimes The Caulbearer stands at the bedroom window and waves until I have rounded the corner, and that pale little face stays in my mind as I weave around cars and pause at red lights. Students fly along pavements on orange scooters, helmets dangling from the handles. Runners trailing earphone wires skirt the perimeter of the Town Moor as the day fades, clouds tinged pink, trees silhouetted against the sky.

4
Hare Moon

Budding Moon, New Shoots Moon,
Seed Moon, Egg Moon, Growing Moon

On the day of the new moon the fields around the town are turning gently yellow. Rapeseed flowers turn their heads to the sun and shiver a little in the spring snow flurries. I remember how these flowers make my aunt sneeze. The patch of grass where we always look out for bunnies is empty today, but there are primroses in the hedgerows, sweet and milky and undeterred by the frost.

That morning, The Littlest One, the one whose face holds the world, woke up and screamed. Her hair clung to her damp chin and her cheeks were smeared with snot. She did not want to get dressed and she did not want to go to school. I held her and rocked her and cajoled her and shushed her while The Caulbearer quietly slipped into her uniform. When The Littlest One feels something, everyone knows it. And now she sits in the back of the car like butter wouldn't melt and I feel a bit ragged but send her a smile through the mirror.

The mornings are brighter now, the sun a little higher in the air. Shadows fall across rooftops as chimneys catch the light and tiles are dappled orange. The sea is a slash of steely blue and I have to force myself to drive back towards the town because the gentle waves are calling me. I would love to run along the coastline watching out for dolphins, or drive out into the hills and lie back on the heather counting clouds, but that must wait.

I have been reading a book by Margaret Hockney, the artist's sister, except that of course she is not just a sister. The book details her career as a nurse and midwife, her travels, her troubled relationship with her mother. I am interested in how the tiny moments in someone's life can get lost, but when pieced together they are something unique and remarkable, how the mundane, repetitive acts add up to a life well lived. I wonder why the gentle, inquisitive actions seem to hold less value, though even as this thought passes through my mind I know I can be a sucker for grand gestures. It's all smoke and mirrors, I know that now, and would pay good money for a decent dose of kindness and calm.

I spend the day in a kind of domestic reverie, dipping in and out of work but distracted by changing beds, stacking the dishwasher, sending emails, tending to my daughter, letting the cat out, making tea, hanging out washing, watering plants, recycling boxes, folding clothes. And all the while I am thinking, weaving ideas in my mind. Someone watching from the outside might see a mother tidying a home, but they would be missing the point. Thoughts are forming, germinating amongst the dirty plates, and they hold more power than people realise.

The Hare Moon is elusive. Evenings are longer, luminous skies reluctant to let go of the day. This moon will be a supermoon, a phenomenon barely visible to the naked eye, but magical none the less, especially when viewed close to the horizon, bobbing on the waves.

Spring seems to be unfolding in a palette of yellow - daffodils that dominated the roadsides a couple of weeks ago are starting to crisp like tissue paper, and I wonder how long it will take for them to die back and make way for summer. Primroses sit in nests of moss, almost too precious to bear, as baby rabbits nibble the grass around them, perilously close to the passing cars. The fields of rapeseed seem cautious this year, tentative and muted as if they can't believe their luck. Hedgerows that were scalped a month or two ago, branches sliced so carelessly their screams echoed across the hills, are fuller and kissed with delicate blackthorn blossom and golden gorse flowers.

The school run feels like a welcome gift each morning. There will often be a tantrum or tears as I unfurl the girls from under their duvets - these breathless moments are rarely completely calm. But once we are in the car, cheeks pink and fairy hair smooth, the landscape works its magic. A kestrel hovering or a buzzard circling on the thermals prompts shouts of excitement, though an owl would be the ultimate prize. Once, The Littlest One spotted a barn owl sitting on a fencepost during the afternoon pickup. I slowed the car and we sat quietly and watched, until the bird twitched its head towards us and unfurled creamy wings, lifting up off the post and flying away over the field like a whisper. For a long time my daughter would ask *where is my barn owl?*, as if the bird had been waiting especially for her, but we have never seen it again.

Once the girls are through the school door I fall into my car, flick on the radio and drive slowly to the top of the hill, where the North Sea is spread in front of me like a banquet. Some days it is a sapphire slick, the stroke of a brush, a sideshow to the castle that perches on the cliffs. Other times the sky becomes the sea and the waves throw up spray that could be clouds. On these days the moisture in the air clings to my face and forms droplets in my hair. Today the sky is the colour of cornflowers and almost completely still. A gentle haze hovers on the horizon, creating a kind of liminal zone between the water and the air. There is frost on the fields, melting into the grass as the sun climbs higher, and the thaw feels like an unfurling in my heart.

It is The Mermaid's birthday. She is fourteen years old, a child in a woman's body. Fourteen years since I pulled this mystical creature from between my legs, out of the water, and stared into her eyes for the very first time. They were dark, fierce and intense, questioning the bright light and the slap of fresh air on her slippery skin - a sensory onslaught. She is a wonder, her brain responding to the universe in ways I still struggle to unravel. Fragile but a warrior, refusing to fall into line with a world that doesn't always hear her, a maypole standing tall as her sisters run around her, trailing ribbons.

I remember the glittering green vest I wore, sparkling like the sea that would later embrace my little girl, as I walked through Peckham following a membrane sweep. It was a week after my due date. Purple stretch marks had started to appear on my abdomen, spreading like wry smiles across the skin. It ached between my legs as I waited for a bus and I looked at people passing by and wondered if they could tell how ripe I was, that my midwife had just felt my baby's head inside my body and how could that even be possible? Such intimacy, another person's fingers stroking my cervix, almost a spell rather than a medical procedure. I wanted to have my baby at home, felt confident in my body's ability to birth my child, and I trusted my midwife to help me to make it happen. I had read Ina May Gaskin's *Guide to Childbirth* and fallen in love with stories involving trusting and waiting.

Sometimes I find it hard to share the pride I felt in birthing my daughters in a pool at home, because so many mothers did not have that experience, and were made to feel less because of it. And this concern over how other women are viewed, the fact that so many women across the world still die in childbirth, the priority of profit over continuity of care, all of this means that I hold my own births tight inside me, afraid to say the wrong thing. Sometimes I feel like an aberration, and in order to sit closely inside the sisterhood I play down my drug-free home births when the topic arises in conversation, and in doing so diminish myself. Even in the moments just after I had held my daughter to my breast, encouraging her to feed so that the placenta would come away, I looked at my husband and gasped *I did it all for you*. As if I was simply an onlooker in my own life, a vessel for everyone else's happiness as well as a traitor to my own sex. This lack of awareness of my own strength and agency, this erosion of self, is the unwanted gift that keeps on giving.

One evening, The Caulbearer crawls into bed to read to me. She is clutching a big book of stories from around the world under her arm. We run our fingers down the contents and find a Buddhist story about a hare and the moon. The hare is wise and tells tales, he is kind and wants happiness for his friends. His generosity is rewarded by the Lord of the Heaven above the Mountain, who dips his finger into rock water and draws the figure of the hare onto the face of the moon. The Caulbearer and I love this story and can't wait for a clear night so we can try to spot the hare.

The Mermaid's legs are getting stronger. She now walks with her great-grandpa's walking stick, preferring the wood that has been smoothed by his hands to the hard edges of crutches. The knocking on her bedroom wall has been replaced by a tap-tap on the floorboards as she makes her way around the house. Emotional connection is important to this daughter. In these last few months of chronic pain she has taken to wearing her Grannie's crystal around her neck and clutching it when she feels distressed. The act of holding it tight in her fist is both a sensory and an emotional necessity, bringing her closer to the safety she craves. I wish I had something to cling on to, because as the outside world slowly opens up, my own world is closing in on me, becoming crowded with more professionals who have opinions on my family and my parenting. When life gets bumpy for a family, it is often the main caregiver who is forced to sit under a burning spotlight, as if that is where the problems originate. My reality is shifting once more and a shell seems to be forming around my heart. I am both raw and numb: nerve endings jangling yet strangely subdued, in a weird process of self-preservation.

My days now involve endless meetings with people who say they are here to help, appearing at my front door with alarming regularity. Today I lead a woman I have never met into the little room next to the kitchen. It is filled with books, jigsaws, *Ikea* storage and a piano, and my four girls are playing with dolls on the carpet. They like to create a world for these dolls, make costumes for them and lose themselves. The visitor has broken that world now, and I look at her, this masked stranger, who has never met my children, who is holding a serious-looking notebook, and I will her to be gentle. Blood is thumping in my ears and there is a sickness in my chest, as the image of my youngest daughter clutching a tiny pair of doll shoes dances behind my eyes.

As the visitor talks, one by one the girls come to me, and I hold them and joke with them and try to do the right thing, because I always try to do the right thing, be a good girl, but somehow life still gets messy. The Mermaid's hands are clawing the carpet as she attempts to stay in the room. Strangers are an issue for her, because there is no history of kindness to reassure her. She has been let down too many times by professionals who promised help but failed to listen. I sit with her, hold her tight as her eyes dart around the room and words choke her throat. Because there are no thoughts that can be voiced. It is enough that her head is filled with horror, and words just make the nightmares more real.

The woman comes through to the lounge with me and we speak for a long time, and when she leaves it is as if the lights in my home have been turned back on. I look at the spider plant hanging its babies over the bookshelf, the picture of my grandmother on her wedding day and the mess of charcoal next to the stove. Familiarity slowly seeps back into my bones and I reclaim my home. The girls have returned to their doll world once more and a small grey cat is mewing at the window, meeting my eyes with her own.

The next Saturday the sky is blue again, split with plane trails but no clouds. The little girls are with their dad and

I have slept for many hours very deeply. When I look in the mirror that morning my face appears smoother, and I am momentarily pleased that sleep can work so efficiently on tired skin.

The Mermaid is keen to swim in our favourite rock-pool, so we drink tea, munch toast and pack bags, taking fluffy dressing gowns and a thermos of tea. An inhaler because the cold water sometimes makes The Mermaid's breaths short and shallow. Swimming costumes under clothes. In the car we suck sherbet lemons, look out for hares and buzzards and fall quiet when we see a deer broken and bloody by the side of the road.

We park up behind the kind of camper van we dream of, with a pop-up roof and a sliding door. The village is throbbing gently with tourists, the beach below speckled with people, weaving between each other like ants on a pavement. Beyond the sand lies a collection of rockpools, hidden behind the lighthouse. Below the lighthouse is a white stag painted onto the rocks. The Mermaid tells me it was painted by Italian prisoners of war during the Second World War, but there is also a legend that a white stag jumped into the sea at that very spot, chased away from nearby Spindlestone, where a princess had been turned into a dragon by a witch. Beautiful and vulnerable or evil and vindictive: there is no middle ground for the women of history, their stories steeped in fear and control. Suddenly the prospect of bathing in the sea feels subversive, an opportunity to reclaim the fairytales and swim through the tears of a dragon.

The Mermaid's lips are dark crimson, which I admire, rarely wearing lipstick myself. I like the way my daughter paints on a face for the waves, but wonder if it is an extension of the mask she often puts on to help her to cope with a world that does not work hard enough to understand her. These rocks, pocked and dented, offer more solace to her than the kind glance of a stranger. There is no subtext, they will always hold pools of salt-water when the tide is low, while wart-like barnacles press sharply into the soles of her feet. She knows the names of all the birds who skitter on the shoreline - sanderlings, redshank and sandpipers. They will never stand so close to her that strange smells invade her nostrils and unsettle her. The birds' staccato chirrups are reassuring, unlike the streams of chatter that pour out of humans, who don't understand that she is silent because she is trying to think and process their words, and so continue to talk to fill the gaps until her head feels like it will explode.

I lay two towels over the cracked limestone, carefully trying to avoid dipping the edges in any residue left by the waves. Our rock pool is spread out just below us, some-how clear and cloudy at the same time. The bottom of the pool is a patchwork of round, flattish stones, while the vertical edges are hung with curtains of kelp, floating like witches' hair.

We shed our clothes and I stand tall in my swimming costume. The air feels surprisingly mild on my bare skin as my daughter leans in to me for support and we walk slowly to the side of the pool. The barnacles and slippery seaweed make it difficult to climb down into the water. We are not brave or stupid enough to jump straight in, submerging ourselves completely: the pale wintery sun of recent months has not yet warmed the sea sufficiently - this is almost the coldest time of year to swim, while frost can still be seen on the windscreens of cars in the early morning - and a sudden dip would steal the breath. Instead, we have learned where natural steps are hidden behind the kelp. We can test the water with our toes, waiting for the burn to spread and skin to turn white. Curious tourists watch from the path, looking at these two figures in swimming costumes with a mixture of surprise and envy. The sanderlings hop and glide behind us, egging us on with their pip-pip-pips.

The Mermaid goes first, gasping as the water reaches her waist and then taking a few frantic strokes, grabbing at the water and bobbing up and down like a puppy. I follow her, sliding off the makeshift step into the icy pool and pushing off a stone with my foot. I glide for a moment, trying to acclimatise and trust my body. Both of us need to swim and then stand, taking minimal respite from the air, which is at least twice as warm as the water. My feet and hands are now stinging and aching, but simultaneously my breath is slowing down and the payoff is beginning. The water feels like oil now, slick and heavy, holding me like it will never let go. The Mermaid is finding it hard to catch her breath, so she crawls up the rock and wraps herself in towels and fluffy dressing gowns, gulping down the Ventolin that will relax the muscles in her airways and allow air into her lungs. Meanwhile, I am in heaven: this is as mindful as it gets for me, wrapped in saltwater with the sun kissing my hair. I feel strong and sensual, and later at home I will wonder what it might be like to swim there with a lover, wrap my legs around his waist and lick the salt from his neck. For now, though, I am thinking of nothing but the smooth pebbles on the cushion of my foot, the resistance of my body against the sea and the endless sky. I swim up and down the pool for about ten minutes, until I can leave my daughter no longer because she is starting to shake and frown. My fingers feel stiff and useless as I grasp the rock and pull myself out of the water, but I stand up, stretching high above the waves, and the salt on my skin feels like armour.

The clouds are suspended like cartoons this evening. I look out of the window on my landing and realise that the view has been blue for as long as I can remember. Tonight though the clouds are three-dimensional, bulging out of the sky like a pop-up book. I walk out of my house and quickly close the front door behind me so the cat doesn't escape. The air is cool and I notice the neighbours' magnolia unfurling its petals. I cross the road and walk a few steps to the corner shop. I need milk for tea, endless tea. Glancing up towards the east, the Hare Moon is translucent and huge. Almost complete, it is only three more days until the full super moon. It is both a source of relief and amazement to me that my heart fidgets and shifts as I stare at the moon, breathing in its glow. It really is a thing, I think. I really am a full moon person, not a new moon person. I am more complete when the moon is as close to a circle as it is possible to be. Less alone. So small and barely visible yet the irony is that I feel bigger. I am baffled, smiling to myself as I push the door and hear the familiar ring of the bell.

In the morning the sky is clear and bright. Across the street a couple are drinking coffee in shirt sleeves. Two sisters, Maggie and Doreen, climb out of their car, one clutching a small black dog. The sisters live just up the road, perhaps a five-minute walk, and every day they visit my neighbour, another sister, at least three or four times. Maggie is as thin as a pin with hair hanging straight and wispy around a pale face with pointed features. She is kind and energetic, always enquiring after The Mermaid. Her shoulders are slightly stooped and she gives the impression of perpetually being one step ahead of the next job. Doreen's features are rounder and bigger, nothing like her sister. Her presence seems clumsy next to neat little Maggie.

I often encounter the sisters on my back lane, where they like to smoke as they lean on the bins. My neighbour, Elsie, doesn't smoke. She has a house that has barely been decorated since she moved into it fifty years ago, all swirling carpets and embossed wallpaper. But it is cleaner than any house on the street. I can plan my year around the domestic chores taking place next door, they are almost as predictable as the cycle of the moon. As spring approaches and the sun rises higher in the sky I know I will bump into Elsie and be reminded of the windows that were installed especially to ensure easier cleaning - *they flip out you see, so they can be reached more easily from the inside.* I will agree that this was a wise decision, as images of my own filthy windows lurk behind my eyes. I will know it is August when I see Maggie and Doreen pulling the surround from a grave out of the boot of a car, and resting it on the floor of the garage to be polished. This grave belongs to Albert, Elsie's husband, and it must be kept as pristine as the home he left behind. The first year I witnessed this event, I stood on my step and wondered what it would be like to miss a man so badly that I would take a cloth and wipe at the dirt of his grave. And then I hated myself for that thought.

The month is dry and dusty. A little pre-summer that reminds me of last year's lockdown, when we sat out on the back lane every day because that was where the sun was. Freckles are forming over noses and I think I look a little less tired. A white band has appeared on my wrist from the watch I wear to time the endless laps of my house.

One evening after school I leave The Mermaid and the two littlest girls with my mum and take The Whirlwind for a bike ride. I run while she cycles ahead, long flaxen hair streaming behind her. We race along a railway path, where the gravel has soaked up the sun, and warm air clings to our skin, forming sweat in pores. Now and then she stops and I run on, until I hear tyres crunching behind me and the bicycle overtakes me once more. We head down the hill towards the river, where stepping stones poke out high above the water line. Turning off the road, I run along a lane of cracked earth and tussocks of brown grass. The Whirlwind is laughing now, because the ground is uneven and when she sings a long note it wobbles around in her throat. In the distance we can see a viaduct, where we will stop for a rest and then turn back. I scan the riverbank for kingfishers. I have seen them here once before, a pair flashing upstream - not today though. Today I trip over the root of a tree, coming so close to falling that my heart rattles around in my chest.

There are a lot of ducks sitting amongst the crops and we watch as a swan glides along the river. The field is huge, and the dusty path that skirts the perimeter reminds me of Languedoc, where I once saw a cloud of hoopoes in a tree. The slow push of the water takes me back to my honeymoon on the Canal du Midi, where we spent long days drinking cheap red wine and playing cards on a tiny boat called Maurice. We slept on a rubber mattress stacked onto a piece of wood on top of the engine. The nights were so hot that our skin would stick to the rubber as the sheet slipped away. It didn't matter that the cabin was airless, we were only breathing each other.

Images of #blossom and #spring have been popping up in my Instagram feed for a couple of weeks now, a premonition of what is to come in Northumberland. As the heat creeps slowly north, warming bark and nudging buds, petals like confetti start to appear in gardens, allotments and on roadsides. The oilseed rape that had seemed so unsure earlier in the month is now vibrant and bold, singing to me on the school run. Hedgerows erupt with birds while rabbits nibble in the sun.

When I look up at the sky, which is blue and cloudless, the outline of evergreen needles and the hazy glare of the light remind me of Bonjour Tristesse. I read that novel for my French A-level and it has stayed with me, tucked inside my soul somewhere, along with memories of grass on bare thighs and stoned Sundays. I read the book just after I realised I loved a boy for the first time. The intensity of those days, those feelings, still fizz in my chest, and several times each year he wanders through my dreams.

The first time I saw him, I had just returned from a French exchange trip, where I really had been immersed in a Sagan novel, rolling around in pine needles with my exchange partner's brother. I was sitting in a pub in town, skin scorched and hair sun-bleached. I felt older than my sixteen years, GCSE results were in and I was heading for sixth form. My friends were clever and just popular enough. They liked smoking in the woods at lunchtime and listening to The Cure, while I sat on the edge of a log and watched. I was never cool, but I was confident on the outside and that got me through.

He was leaning on the bar, Diesel jacket, fair hair in tight curls. He turned to look at my table and I caught his eye. Or maybe he caught mine. He smiled and turned back and I knew I would kiss him someday soon. He was the farmer's son, a small time weed dealer. Cheeky and charming and his freckled face was soft under my lips.

The first time he came back to my house, my mother walked in to find him sprawled in the kitchen and saw exactly what was happening and how it would end, but she had to just watch from the sidelines while I loved him. And for a time he loved me too, picking me up from school in his brown Mini Metro and leaving his townie friends behind to collect me from theatre rehearsals.

His family's farm was a few miles from the market town where I lived, up a hill, past the old racecourse and along winding roads that made me giddy. The single storey farmhouse, built new sometime in the eighties maybe, was nothing like the knackered grandeur of my own house, and his family thought I was posher than I was. We probably looked and spoke like we had inherited our ramshackle home, but really we were just chasing a dream.

My parents had fallen in love with a mustard monstrosity that was built in the seventeenth century and grew over the years. A sash window here, a marble fireplace there. The house was huge, a three-storey box built into the hill that took me to the farm. Everyone in the town thought my family was fancy because of that house, and because of my dad's sweary rogueishness that was delivered with more than a hint of public school. In 1988 it was possible to buy a big pile of bricks in the countryside for a reasonable sum if you searched hard enough and didn't mind a project. My parents had started in Devon and looked at houses further and further north as they tried to outrun the ballooning housing market. They attempted a ruined beauty in Sheffield but it was completely uninhabitable and there were four children to think of. My mum fell in love with a picture perfect cottage in Derbyshire, but the chocolate box wasn't to be: too expensive and her husband was still dreaming of castles in Scotland. They settled in Yorkshire, in the mustard house with a broken roof that would swallow almost every penny.

I had a bedroom at the very top of the house, in the furthest corner. It was nearly as big as the ground floor of my home now, with a black Victorian fireplace and a dual aspect. The house had once been a school, and this was where the headmistress had slept. The bay window looked out over the town, where a flag fluttered at the top of the castle and cobbles tumbled down towards the river. On the other side of the room there was another window, with a wooden seat from where I would curl up and gaze into the garden. There was a huge copper beech that I would climb with my younger brothers and sister, and vegetable beds that crawled up to an ancient red brick wall. You could climb some stone steps to an outside space that my mum optimistically called 'the art studio', but was essentially a dusty room where children could hide and mothers could dream.

My room was sliced in half horizontally with a floral border, and I painted the walls pink above and green below in an act of half-hearted teenage rebellion. When the farmer's son visited he would give me mix tapes from a house club in Blackpool called *Zone*, and I would play them on a blue ghetto blaster from Boots I was given for my eleventh birthday. I developed a diet of house music and musical theatre, with a hint of breathy St Etienne pop and 60s girl bands thrown in for nostalgia. My friends were all into indie music, but it felt too dark for me, I needed to feel a little closer to the light. I leaned heavily on music as a prompt for the emotions forever bubbling dangerously under my skin, even creating a mix tape entitled 'Sad Songs For Crying', in case life wasn't enough to tip me into tears.

I always felt like an outsider, but now I am older I wonder whether that outside feeling is just a normal girl feeling. A trying to fit into a world for men feeling. A scared to say what you think unless it's wrong feeling. A how do I make people smile feeling. A why do I care so much and what if they laugh at me feeling. Whatever it is, it's a tough feeling to shake.

The confused summer weather finally breaks. The supermoon that we had all anticipated is a washout in our little corner of the world. Newspapers and social media are full of hazy pink moons like balls of candyfloss throbbing above Stonehenge and the Golden Gate Bridge. In Northumberland there is only cloud. Slowly I am learning from the moon how to deal with disappointment, but also how to hope. Tonight the sky is a shadow of what could have been, but tomorrow might be another story.

A couple of nights earlier, having read about the predicted weather, I step out of the house with The Whirlwind dressed in a dog onesie and cross the street, barefoot. We turn and look beyond our roof at the sky, which is smug and dreamy, luxuriating in the glow of the almost-full moon. All week the moon has been brilliant - bold and bossy, leaning in on my world. Standing on tarmac with gravel between my toes, holding my daughter's hand, which is rough and dry from too much washing, I breathe and smile. *I don't see the moon in a spiritual way mummy*, says The Whirlwind, *I just look at the craters and think of the science*. And that's it right there: all the thoughts I have are attached to emotions. A friend describes me as a romantic to her realist. I would love to explain everything away with scientific theory, but I've always been a dreamer so the facts just don't make sense on their own.

As the Hare Moon hides behind curtains of rain, I pull down my blind and bury myself in phone calls from occupational therapists and physios, appointments with a psychiatrist, warnings from an education welfare officer and meetings with therapists. And all the while The Mermaid is floundering. I am trying to hold her tight but she is slipping from my grasp and the waves are pulling her away. Friends tell me that I seem distant, that I am isolating myself. And they mean well but I don't know how not to hide, like the moon submerged in gloom. It is enough for me to hold everything in my frazzled mind tightly tightly tightly so the horror doesn't seep out. My therapist's emails sit unanswered in my inbox. The very last thing I need right now is someone mirroring my words, highlighting them so they flash brightly like a billboard.

That night, I dream that my cat is swirling in icy water, fur sticking up in wet peaks, eyes terrified. I can't reach her, and the cat keeps disappearing below the surface because the current is so strong. When I wake up the cat is drinking from the glass next to my bed, *sup sup sup*, and my throat is raw and painful when I swallow. I let her out while I go into the kitchen to make a cup of tea. Slowly a thrum grows louder from the utility room: it is raining onto the plastic roof. As the sugar dissolves into my tea I return to the front door, where the cat sits, dripping. I close the door on the weather as a wet tail brushes against my leg.

It's another weekend where I must drive the three youngest girls down to their dad's and pretend it doesn't hurt. I remind myself that the alternative was unsustainable but the empty bunk beds are hard to bear. It's not that I don't want my children to see their father, or that I can't see the benefit of things he can offer that I can't. It is the enforcedness of it all, the way I must relinquish control and be told that this is how it is. The fact that I can't hold my daughters even if I want to, and they can't hold me, because this weekend it is not allowed. I leave my phone on all night, because I have promised The Caulbearer I am always here. *You can always call me and I will come.*

The previous night The Caulbearer couldn't sleep. She was quiet and her eyes dipped down under long lashes. It was the night before she went away and I knew she was full of conflict and confusion, between loving and leaving. I lifted my duvet and pulled her in, holding her tightly and feeling skinny knees digging into my legs. I told her that even when we are apart, my heart is always full of the girls and they are always on my mind. Love doesn't stop just because you can't see it, the moon is always there even on a cloudy night. Words tumbled from my mouth in a waterfall of clichés, but I believed them all and maybe they are clichés because they are true. My tears dripped into her hair but a little cry did us both good and this is why my phone is always on.

While they are away, I write and I read and I swim and I try to stop The Mermaid's legs from trembling, holding them and stroking them to find that elusive calm. The sun shines and the rain pours and all the time the blossom is falling from the trees and the moon is shrinking.

On the Saturday night, The Mermaid isn't well. I know when it is about to happen, when my daughter will slip out of the present and become trapped in a nightmare. Her eyes will start to flicker and her wrist contorts. Her entire body is alert, taut. Sometimes her lips move, terrified, almost-whispers pour out of her mouth in a staccato rhythm. I can never pull her back from the brink in time: the other world holds too much power. I can only sit and stroke and tell my daughter that she is safe, until the moment passes and suddenly she will slump against my shoulder, exhausted and confused. It's as if a demon has been exorcised. And then The Mermaid talks. She empties her head of the shadows and it feels like too much for me to hold. I tuck her into bed, soothed by a hot water bottle and the knowledge that her mother is next door. And then I lie in my bed with a heart full of acid and a head swimming with ghosts.

There are three empty beds tonight, the house feels cold. There will be no sleep. I pad out of my room, across the landing towards the bathroom where the waning Hare Moon is hanging strangely low in the sky, bright as an eye. I lean over my plants to take a closer look, and that is when I see it, imprinted into the glow, a hare lifting its head towards the stars.

5
Mother's Moon

*Milk Moon, Bright Moon, Hare Moon,
Grass Moon*

Dunstanburgh Castle looks like an upside-down cow, jagged hooves licked by the salt spray blown off the North Sea, flank wedged into the grassy turf. I tried to swim here once, in a cove that could only be reached by limbo-dancing under a fence and scrambling down very steep rocks, but the swirling current was too strong. This exposed headland between the villages of Embleton and Craster has been occupied since prehistoric times. The history books write of battles and warriors, but shards of pottery, Roman brooches and hearths that were unearthed in the 1920s reassure me that women's voices once floated across the marram grass too.

As the Hare Moon wanes for the last time and the Mother's Moon prepares to dazzle, I drop the two littlest girls at their dance class and head to the beach below the castle to fill the hour with a swim. The Mermaid and I have been swimming regularly now as her legs grow stronger, and strip down to our costumes, acclimatised to

77

the icy burn. But The Whirlwind is unconvinced and creeps onto the sand in a wetsuit that is too big. The sky is grey, like a piece of cotton wool wiping away a smoky eye. Two men sit on folding chairs behind fishing rods and we walk on a little further to avoid being snagged by their lines.

A strange, fizzing energy is bubbling on the shoreline, scratching at the sand and sending terns smashing into the waves. The tide is fairly high, and conceals a slope on the beach that means we are in up to our waist after only a few wincing steps. Grains of sand twist under the balls of my feet as the current wraps water tightly around my legs. I have not known the sea to be this fierce before, relentless and pounding. We like to swim in on a wave just before it breaks, but somehow these waves keep crashing on top of us, however we position ourselves in the water. The Mermaid is bounced off the sand and emerges spluttering, red lipstick still perfectly intact. Moments later, I misjudge my dive and roll over and over, eyes squeezed shut so I don't lose my contact lenses. I'm lung-punched but exhilarated and float on my back beyond the breakers, just in time to see a wetsuited Whirlwind collide with a huge wave and jump up screaming in terror. She is hysterical and furious, railing at the sea and matching its temper. I laugh at her drama and it feels like I am looking in the mirror, fire matching fire.

Later that evening I take her hand, and we pad in our dressing gowns onto the street. There is no sign at all of the Mother's Moon and the sky is still a smudge, clouds in ribbons trailing through the sky. But we know it is there, we felt it in the tides, nipping at our ankles. It is always there.

The Caulbearer is in a funny mood, refusing to speak, brow all scrunched and furrowed, replying *I don't know* to every question I ask. At bedtime, she and The Littlest One climb up onto my bed dressed as a tiger and a sheep in their onesies. This is one of my favourite parts of the day, when I can lie down and do all the voices in the bedtime stories. We are on the last Harry Potter book and it's sinister. I am grateful that the sky is as peachy pink as the roses on my windowsill because I'm delivering a scene where Voldemort is torturing a witch suspended by her ankles from the ceiling. And there is a snake - The Caulbearer has a thing about snakes and I can feel her tense little body pushing hard into my ribs as the scene unfolds. I do all the accents - I must do all the accents because if I forget that Professor McGonagall is Scottish they make me start the paragraph again.

Tonight I am exhausted. My brain feels like it is being squeezed and twisted, as if someone is forcing grains of sand through a timer and speeding the world up. When I finish the chapter I would normally scoop the little girls up and pop them into bed, before starting to settle the older two. But I am warm under the duvet with my tiger and my sheep, and I say *let's stay in here and cuddle*, so they nuzzle into my neck.

When I was pregnant the last time, I invented the Story Room. I was juggling part-time teaching with home education, and the days were defined by mothering and trying to cling on to an identity separate from my children. I was still breastfeeding The Caulbearer, until she told me my milk tasted funny and stopped just like that. It's not true what they tell you about breastfeeding being a contraceptive. I dreamed this fourth baby into existence, but by this stage I had no idea how we would manage until death us do part. I was spinning with girls, giddy with all the mothering, but there was a void somewhere that was bigger than all of us.

After lunch each day, with crumbs on the breadboard and pieces of apple turning brown under the high chair, I would tell the girls it was time for The Story Room, a magical place full of books and cushions, where sunbeams dance off the ceiling. The four of us would traipse up the stairs, creaking under our combined weight, and finger the spines of the books in the scuffed bookcase, wondering which ones would make it into the Story Room today. As dust danced in the light, we would curl under the duvet of my bed, heels and elbows nudging me from inside and out, as we drifted between worlds, sometimes asleep, other times awake. And this is what happens again on an exhausted Monday evening: a tiger and a sheep on each shoulder and a doze underneath a kaleidoscope sky.

Later that night, when the little girls are back in their own beds and I am playing Scrabble with The Mermaid and The Whirlwind on a knitted blanket, I spy a skinny moon from my bedroom window for the first time. We lean our cheeks against the cold glass and stare. I have never seen the moon from this position before and I fall back onto the pillows holding my oldest girls tight. My breathing is slow and deep, and this moon and I make a pact. I am not looking to her for solace, imploring her with my eyes as my soul breaks in two, it's not that sort of evening. But there's an awareness, a mutual respect. That night I sleep with my blind open.

I have been taking Sertraline for a couple of years. I was prescribed it by my GP to tackle my anxiety around the time my universe broke. Since I was ten years old my anxiety has manifested as Obsessive Compulsive Disorder during times of intense stress - my busy, neurotic brain is a perfect breeding ground for obsessional thoughts. In 1987 no one had heard of OCD. There were no websites with cartoon characters spouting child-friendly wisdom in speech bubbles. School nurses did not sit in a small room helping you to unravel the horror. Child mental health was not a thing. I just washed and washed my hands and counted in threes while the shame soaked into my bones.

OCD is all about control, or lack of control. The world is spinning off its axis and the only way to moor it is to listen to the voices in your head that deliver clear and repetitive instructions. Not actual voices, I have never been psychotic, but there is a vicious narrative pulsing along my neural pathways when OCD rears its head. It feels like an unwelcome but familiar visitor. A kind of toxic co-dependency develops between me and the OCD and it is very hard to end the relationship.

Shame is the most debilitating aspect of OCD, the way it can convince you that you are both completely powerless and a monster. I bumbled along for years, not noticing that my OCD was worse when I was scared, when life was unpredictable and when I was exhausted. It was only after The Caulbearer was born, when I was thirty-five, that I started to really pay attention to what was happening inside my mind.

2012 was a perfect storm for my OCD: my husband was working long hours, trying to build a business from scratch; school and my oldest daughter did not get along; I gave birth to my third daughter; seven weeks later we moved to the house between the hills and the sea.

The day we got the keys to the new house, to this house I am in now, I stood in one of the bedrooms next to the baby Caulbearer, who dozed in a car seat on the carpet. I looked onto the back lane, tiled rooftops joined up like a jigsaw, TV aerials slicing the skyline, and I wondered what would happen next.

What happened next was that I fell to pieces.

It all came to a head when I had to tax the car and there was nowhere to park outside the post office. Such a silly thing. I scooted onto a yellow line and left The Mermaid and The Whirlwind inside the car with the window a tiny bit open because I know you never leave a child in the car and if you do then you must open a window. And they sat good as gold, reading books as I strapped The Caulbearer to my chest and dashed into the post office. I was in there for maybe five minutes, popping my head out every 30 seconds to check the girls and make sure I didn't have a ticket. And the last time I came out, with a receipt for my car tax and a baby's sweaty cheek against my chest, a woman and her husband were standing next to my car looking very cross. The woman was about my mum's age but she was definitely not my mum. She told me she had been timing me and watching my children who were far too young to be left in a car, and what was I thinking? My legs were straight away jelly and I felt sick in my throat. I started to explain that I had just moved here and I didn't know anyone who could help me and I had to tax the car and my baby needed feeding and the girls were fine they were just reading and they knew where I was and I had been checking on them. But the woman's eyes bore into me and her face was stern and pinched. She thought I was a bad mother, and she tutted and walked away.

Not long after that, while I was trying hard to be a good mother, tucking in the duvet on The Whirlwind's new bunk bed, an insect scuttled across the whiteness of the sheet, under the duvet and into the darkness, and my OCD told me that it was a bedbug. For weeks after that, I googled 'bedbugs' and checked and checked the beds and the sofas for evidence that they had infested our house. I checked my body and my children's bodies for bites, and on one particularly dark night I took a torch and shined it under my daughter's duvet as she slept, because Google told me that they came out at night and that was how you could confirm their presence.

Night times were a horror film. I was convinced my mattress was full of creatures and was awake most of the night feeding my beautiful new baby girl who I had to protect from the non-existent bugs. Any tickle against my leg or mark on my sheets required a full inspection. My breath hovered high up in my chest as I fell into an uneasy sleep, and when I opened my eyes each morning I gave thanks for the brief respite before it all started again.

Funny that the parking ticket woman broke the camel's back. Under the Mother's Moon, I read a book, Little Bandaged Days, about a mother's descent into madness. Her reality slowly merges into a paranoia, an alternative universe that I can recognise. And I wonder if madness is really madness at all, or just the brain's way of coping with extreme stress, like a filter that has become blocked, or a filing system that is broken. The woman in the book has a husband that works all the hours too, a madness that grows out of an absence.

When you are living in a removed reality, call it madness if you like, time takes on a very dangerous quality. Every moment is precarious. Minutes fly out of your hands like trapped butterflies, only to flutter behind your back and re-emerge as something quite different. The ability to navigate time is reduced to robotic routines. I would sit at the kitchen table each morning and write down a small list of essential jobs just so I could feel a pang of hope when I crossed one off. That tiny stroke of biro kept the bedbugs at bay for another five minutes, but the obsessive thoughts and compulsive checking had started to be swallowed by a heaviness that the health visitor called post-natal depression.

I wasn't used to depression, this total winding down of the clock. Everything about me was a hundred miles an hour, not this leaden-limbed woman with sad eyes that didn't match her smile. Holding The Mermaid's hand as I traipsed across the park, pushing a buggy and cradling a small baby's head under my chin, my feet felt like weights that would drag me down through the grass, deep into the mud that crawled with worms and roots that would wrap their tendrils around me and keep me there. One morning I wore my wellies over pyjama bottoms and spent many days after that feeling the burn of my cheeks as I trudged past perfectly manicured mums at the school gate. Terrible, the power of shame, the way it seeps into your soul and claims a home.

After several weeks of imaginary bedbugs and inadequate lists, my madness had started to become an inconvenience, interrupting the daily routine. Luckily for us all, a few sessions of NHS cognitive behavioural therapy and maybe just good old-fashioned time seemed to do the trick. Relative calm was restored and my madness was no longer getting in the way.

A few years later when my OCD resurfaced, when all the safety nets had been ripped to shreds and the only thing that remained was medication, Sertraline kept the bedbugs away. *You're on a homeopathic dose* said the GP scathingly, but it seemed to help somehow, if only by creating a twice-daily ritual of water down the throat and my own eyes staring back at me in the bathroom mirror.

Two years on I have become an expert at administering medication to The Mermaid, two pills in the morning, two in the evening and painkillers as required. I am so focused on giving her the correct dose that I keep forgetting to take my own medicine. And then the GP says I have to have an appointment before they can prescribe me any more and I can't get an appointment that suits me or leave the house anyway. So I stop taking the Sertraline.

My temper shortens a little, and my nerve-endings need less of a tug to get a reaction. For a few nights I wake with a jolt, hearing mice that aren't there or an imaginary murderer creaking up my stairs. And I feel raw. More exposed than when I fling myself onto a wave and crash onto the sand. Tears threaten to spill over several times each day and somehow everything is more vicious yet also achingly beautiful.

I live a life in micro fashion that lurches from crisis to crisis but is largely unobserved by the outside world. Just like mothering is micro because so many people do it but no one talks about what it really means. Like an avalanche, it only takes one stone to tumble before the whole thing collapses. Society likes families to fit neatly into boxes, everything in its place, and when they look slightly different, well, that's when things can get really messy. I'm living life on high alert: always quickly trying to catch the next falling stone, constantly holding my children's emotions, trying to set them free but delicately keeping them safe. Shrugging off comments on my parenting or the way I should have behaved as a wife as if they are water off my tired back. It's all white noise that you forget is there until it suddenly stops. And you break. I break.

It is the night the Mother's Moon becomes whole. A lunar eclipse is occurring, creating a reddish glow as the Earth's umbral shadow covers the moon. I am watching the sky as I sit at my desk. The movement of smoky cloud shifting across the sky is hypnotic, hints of light glowing behind the swirls. Every now and then a patch of blue reveals itself, a little tease.

I wonder if my sister can see the Mother's Moon bathed in blood from the wicker chair on her stoop on the other side of the world. We have been texting this morning, missing each other, and there is no date in the diary when we might next hold each other because the borders are still closed.

She ran away to New Zealand when she was still a child-woman. It was never really clear to me what she was looking for: maybe she saw herself in the vibrant Pohutakawa trees, treasured by Maoris for their strength and beauty. With a face full of freckles that invites people in, my sister's brown eyes tell a million stories depending how the light hits them. Crazy Cathy Corby. All or nothing. Living at a hundred miles an hour then crashing to a halt. Like the wind that whips Wellington's harbour, there is rarely a lull. Australia claimed her in the end.

I like to think of her on her porch, amongst the road-side treasures she has collected - Grecian urns, wooden chairs and yucca plants; my niece curled onto her lap, long legs like her grandad tucked up; my nephew, face sprinkled with his mother's freckles, crouched in the yard cuddling the guinea pigs. Sometimes in the evenings, when I stand barefoot on my own step and look for the moon, I am comforted by the thought that the sun is shining on my sister.

Another professional appears at the front door, face covered in a black mask, but I think (hope?) there is kindness in her eyes. I hover by the kettle while she fires questions at my children. After a few minutes she asks to speak to me on her own and the younger three melt away onto the back lane while The Mermaid floats upstairs.

We sit in the lounge. There are pictures on the wall in there, given to me by my husband, and I am momentarily grateful that I can look at them without my stomach lurching. I sit on the very edge of the sofa facing the visitor, who is making notes in her big black notebook. My face is pale. I have been crying on and off while the girls were at school and I am thin in the way that excessive stress makes you thin - full of an empty that no one can see.

Earlier I texted my husband to ask him something about our divorce. The messages went back and forth and back and forth until I remembered I could never feel satisfied after these exchanges, only smashed to pieces. This is why I can feel my hip bones and why my freckles stand out on translucent skin.

Before the messages and the smashing to pieces I was researching and discussing medication for The Mermaid. I was writing down the times of her appointments this week with a psychiatrist and a therapist. I was speaking on the phone to an education specialist and trying to explain again why my daughter finds formal learning absolutely terrifying. And then I cried.

And before all of that, early this morning I woke the two youngest girls for school, laying out their uniforms on the radiator in their bedroom. I stroked their hair and pulled up the blind to reveal a rain-lashed window. The Littlest One rubbed sleepy eyes and smiled, while The Caulbearer scowled at me and slammed a door against her sister. And then she ignored me at breakfast, on the school run and even when I kissed the top of her head like I always do as the teacher opened the door. More tears (mine).

This is the backdrop to where I am now, sitting on the edge of my sofa. She has caught me when I am vulnerable, this visitor, and my guard is down. She talks about procedures and support and *what do you think is best*, and my brain starts to burn, leaking behind my eyes until tears threaten to spill again and I just want it all to stop. And it is three years ago again, and my hip bones rub even more against my jeans, my face a cheap Munch, cheeks sunken and eyes haunted. Hunted. I step out of myself and I watch this woman on the sofa, scared and intimidated and exhausted and I think who is she? Where has she come from? And the common denominator is the elephant in the room, the pictures hanging in front of me. When I redecorated this room after he left I thought I had brushed away the anger, the indifference and the hurt. Yet somehow they have resurfaced under the daubs and that is why there is a woman bent over sobbing on a couch. She has not managed to erase him as successfully as she had hoped.

As the full moon approaches, I receive pictures on my phone of a burning red orb suspended over my sister's house. There are palm trees and dusty footpaths, Willie Wagtails nesting under the tiles on the neighbour's roof. She texts me *night night* and I am impatient to catch the moon when it rises here because there is a chance she can still see it and that means we are closer somehow.

After school I take the two littlest girls to a class with my dancer friend on a cricket pitch. While they make mosaics out of flowers and spin under the trees, I head to Dunstan Steads for a brief reunion with a friend and a scream in the surf. I have not seen this friend for a couple of years. When we talk we complete each other's thoughts and the words pour fast and furious. I spot her in the marram grass on a sand dune, tucked snugly into a wetsuit and watching the waves smashing onto the beach, churning gold as grains of sand are whipped into a frenzy. We run towards each other across the sand and cling on. She is wild too, this friend, her ferocity often carefully concealed under a sweet nature and a sprinkling of self-doubt. I love her smiling eyes and her open mind, and today she is unfazed by the branches of seaweed being tossed onto the shore, and the diagonal waves roaring at us.

The cloud is stubborn and I imagine the supermoon will show itself only in the tides. Stripped down to my costume, I throw myself into the breakers, occasionally scratching my skin on the sand or tasting salt on my tongue. The Mermaid and my friend dance in the froth, while her husband laughs and videos the sea witches. For a time I am right in the middle of the moment, far away from the crises currently punctuating my existence. My body is pawed and clawed and ravished and licked and this is what I needed. This is why I was so confused by the woman sobbing on the sofa, knackered and fractured, when look at her now, she is everything.

Another day, another appointment. The sun has got his hat on but there's no time to play. I try to distract my crowded head by doing some very mundane jobs. With three kids safely in their classrooms and The Mermaid still sleeping, I wrestle the hoover from underneath a pile of bikes in the utility room and drag it out of the front door. I have leased a boring new family car and it is already soaked in sand and bits of grass. I have vowed to keep it nice for as long as possible, and the girls tell me I always say that but this time I might try to mean it.

I am attempting to suck the anxiety out of my brain and ground myself, looking for areas of my life I still have some control over. Some of the sand is going up the hoover, but a lot of stubborn grains have become snarled up in the upholstery of the car and they won't shift. My brain is mashed and clumsy analogies are swimming around my head.

I heave the hoover back inside, feeling no more in control and a little more desperate. A fat pigeon is sitting on our bird feeder, looking pathetically at the water in the bowl that has turned slightly green. I flick the kettle on in a familiar ritual and miss the gritty-eyed dark mornings when it was just me and the cat and the rest of the world could wait. Reach into the cupboard where I keep all the pills. As I pull the medication out of the cupboard, I notice a small sealed plastic bag, right at the back, containing a herbal remedy. A couple of years ago, running out of ways to bring her back to me, I took The Mermaid to see a herbalist. I press out a couple of tablets that are definitely stronger than anything the herbalist gave us. During the time when no one listened and no one understood my daughter she kept getting sicker and sicker until I had to accept that the herbs were not working. I pour boiling water on some orange juice, and take it upstairs with the medication.

While she wakes I send a couple of emails, fold some clothes, make my bed, unstack and restack the dishwasher and put on a load of washing. I'm on autopilot, roboti-cally creating the impression of a home that is organised and cared for in the hope that it will conceal my frazzled mind.

I nip up to the allotment, gutted to see that while I have neglected it over the last rainy fortnight, it has turned into a jungle. The tulips have shed their petals and been replaced by bluebells and dandelion clocks. There is rhubarb, I notice, a few red onions. Endless blossom and thistles. No time to stop though, because I have thought of another area of my life I can control: my tiny front lawn that I can mow. Back down the lane, pulling the lawn mower behind me, over the road, where the postman is dashing between doorways. The cat is waiting at the door. She looks at me scathingly, knows I'm not up to much.

I'm vaguely aware that I am supposed to be a full moon person. Today I should be feeling fulfilled and energised, but instead I am sterile and empty and still the moon is nowhere to be seen.

It's half term and the sun is shining hard. Except on the beaches, where a sea fret lingers like steam from a train. Across Facebook and on my own street, all the talk is of this fog that has cast an icy spell over coastal Northumberland, as if it is not a phenomenon that occurs in the North-East every year.

I have promised to take The Mermaid for a swim, but as we drive out of town the trees are barely visible and the temperature on the gauge in the car drops by several degrees. There can be no swimming today in this chilly mist, so I turn the car around, noting The Mermaid's alarm at the change in plans and hoping the fret won't follow us.

Our allotment is still bathed in sunshine, and the girls spend the rest of the afternoon playing explorers and locking each other in the shed. The sky is a violent blue, like something is about to happen. I dig over a grotty bit of soil where the trampoline used to live and start to roll out pieces of turf to extend the lawn. Sun burns into my neck and mud clags my nails. There's a small satisfaction in the digging and the pulling of weeds, the knowledge that I am moulding this land. I tread hard onto the turf with my old trainers, trying to flatten out the bumps, lifting it up at the edges and pushing bits of soil into the dips. It's not a thing of beauty, my lawn, but it's good for handstands and dens.

When we were first offered this allotment, it was full of fruit trees, vegetable gardens and beautifully weeded flower beds. Almost immediately I dug over a large area of soil and spent a wet Saturday morning laying turf down. In those days, Saturdays used to involve very early mornings and vinyl, a man in his dressing gown taking records in and out of sleeves and stacking them up on the floor. There was a baby gym, but I can't remember which baby, and an *Ikea* high chair that would catch my toe when I walked past. Much later I would find the tops of beer bottles under the decks, fliers from old club nights, and my stomach would hurt. The music was good though.

Now and then I feel a huge sense of overwhelm about our massive allotment and a pang of guilt that it's a bit messy, and this will often coincide with a turfing frenzy. I can leave the grass to the moths and the bees, watch thistles spear the apple blossom and keep one bed for vegetables and another for flowers. When the weather's good and The Mermaid feels up to it, I spend a lot of time up here, pulling weeds and pottering about. I make a mug of tea in my kitchen and take it across the road so I can sip it in the sun. I'll perch on one of the old stakes that marks the edge of the veg bed and listen to the tap tap tap of my neighbour's walking stick on the lane. He always remarks on how good the weather is. That's what people do up here.

A couple of days later the sun has burned the fog away, though it glares at us from the horizon. We decide to head to our favourite rock pool. The hedges are full of blackthorn blossom and chaffinches, and the rapeseed looks like egg yolk. I stop at the level crossing and fiddle with my phone, looking for music. Reggae is sunny music and Johnny Osbourne shows up in my album list. The sound quality is scratchy and lazy, like the record we used to listen to, and it's a relief it doesn't hurt to hear it. I can sing along without breaking my heart and it's just part of the soundtrack of my life. The barriers go up and I run a little scenario in my head, telling Lauren Laverne why this is one of my Desert Island Discs. The girls try to identify the cheeky horns and suck on sherbet lemons.

Bamburgh is full of extended families and I don't see anyone who looks like me. I don't see any other women on their own with four children. No one looks like a person in their own right. They all look like mothers, or fathers, or grandparents, or children, or groups of friends, or young couples, or second time married baby boomers. I watch them carefully and wonder who they are, what they are doing. What is your tragedy I wonder? Is your heart smashed to a pulp? Do you lie awake wondering how to stop your children from hurting? Do you read articles in the paper and want to talk about them over endless cups of tea but there is no one there? Do you stop and think about your life and wonder what happened? Do you look in the mirror and wish someone knew your face as well as you do? Wish that someone wanted to stroke it and know every freckle? Can you see all of this when you look at me in my family car with my four daughters? Or maybe I'm missing something and you are wearing your mask just like me, careful not to let it slip and reveal a sorrow too painful to share. Perhaps you look at me and see a warrior striking out against the odds, gifted beyond belief to be wrapped in four sweet girls.

But no one looks at me. Until we park the car and the girls run down the grassy slope towards the rocks. Until I spread towels over the barnacles, pour the little ones into wetsuits and roll orange armbands up their arms. Until a sea witch emerges from under an oversized woollen jumper and lowers herself into the bladderwrack that floats up from the sides of the pool, and wetsuited children cling to her neck as she glides through the water. And then they look. They stand with their walking jackets and their dogs, eating ice creams and watching gannets through binoculars. They stare at this family in the icy sea and the sea witch challenges them with her eyes.

One of the girls says *why is everybody staring Mummy?* And I tell them it is because we are a tribe of girls and perhaps they want a little piece of our magic.

The Mother's Moon is waning but you would never know. I have not seen it for many days. Summer is rushing in, I can smell it in the heat of the pavements and the lilac in the air. I can stare at the sky from my bed when I am reading to the girls at night and we are distracted by the light show. A tangerine glow beyond the rooftops is seamlessly sliced by trails of cloud that burn pink. When the world was locked down the sky became my best form of entertainment. I wasn't sure then, and I'm still not sure now, why it took me so long to look up. Too busy trying to quell my itchy feet. When I feel trapped by circumstance, the fleeting nature of clouds, the shape-shifting absorbs me and I can fly a million miles while I'm standing still. The view from my window can take me out of my head as much as the stories I read to my children every night.

One evening, just before bed, I open the front door to call the cat in. As I whistle softly she shoots into the garden from behind me and a daughter tells me the cat was asleep on the bunk bed all along. Now she has a taste of freedom and will not be coaxed back in with biscuits. She can't believe her luck, strutting down towards the lane with her tail bouncing.

This is an irritation. I have a new book on the go, fresh sheets on my bed and a deep desire to be lying in it. If the cat stays out all night The Mermaid and her sisters will worry. I will worry a little bit too, not just because I love the cat, but because if anything happens to her I am scared it will be the very last straw for our family. Also she will miaow really loudly outside my bedroom window at 3 a.m. and wake me up.

I call to the girls that I am going to fetch the cat in, slip socked feet into sandals and lock the front door behind me. At the far end of the street the horizon is burning red beyond the town. A man is sitting in the window of a house looking down at his phone. He doesn't look at me. That's part of the problem of living in a small town in the middle of nowhere. Everyone sees me, but no one really looks.

I am calling the cat's name softly, pebbles on the lane dusty under my sandals. The birdsong is intense for so late I think. It's dusk now, surely they should all be in their nests. I look over the fence at the allotments, watching for a movement that might indicate my cat. A big ginger tom saunters through a gate but no grey tabby.

Earlier that day I pranged my expensive and boring new family car just near this spot. I could feel the *I told you so* in the kids' expressions. I misjudged the corner, squeezing and scratching the hub against a parked van.

My car came off worse, dented and scraped, while my neighbour's van didn't feel a thing. I was rushing, always rushing, and I am cross with myself for doing it but there is no time to worry about it now, maybe I won't see how close I am to dropping all the balls if I just keep moving.

It is this van that my cat now pops out from behind, before promptly darting up the back lane. I sigh and follow her, and something flits past the corner of my eye. The cat startles and gets ready to pounce. Another flit, and I recognise the delicate flap of wings. Bats on my back lane. As my eyes grow accustomed to the gloom, I can see that there are more, dipping under the washing lines that hang between the houses. My dad called for bats with a click click click of his tongue in the garden where I got married, and I think of him now as they dive around my head. Remember him standing on the lawn, wine glass in one hand while we laughed and strained our eyes in the darkness, just before I became a bride.

The cat will not be caught and I need to go back to the children. When I step inside The Caulbearer is sitting on the stairs asking *where is the cat*? I tell her all about the night-time excitement and she jumps up in her zebra pyjamas and dots out of the house onto the pavement, just in time for a bat to dance through the beam of a street lamp. And together we shake biscuits and count bats and wonder where the moon has gone, until a little striped cat trip-traps into the house and I can turn the key and go to bed.

*   *   *

At the end of the half term holiday I take the three young-est girls camping in the Lake District, leaving The Mermaid with my parents. I want to see fells towering above me, walk until my hips are aching and my skin is scorched, and The Mermaid will not manage that. I have not left her for over six months, but my parents are her favourite people outside of our house, and the little ones and I need an adventure.

The night before we drive to Ullswater, my mum looks after the girls while my dad and I sing with their local choir. The gift of song from my mum. Dad and I drive to a quarry a few miles out of town because we must sing where our potentially lethal breath will float away over the treetops. The air is muggy, a sky pregnant with clouds threatening rain that never shows. Turning off the main road, we cross over a stone bridge. Everything is verdant and expectant. Pulling into a makeshift car park above the quarry, the air is fizzing with midges and dust disturbed by tyres. A wooden portacabin is decorated with coloured tiles and saplings have been planted nearby. The choir's conductor stands on the edge of a clearing, where a wire runs from a keyboard along the path. A circle of stones and tree stumps are surrounded by birdsong and I wander off to look at huge bulrushes while my dad finds himself in a conversation about Cervantes and feminism with a visiting musician.

I have a high soprano voice, not much vibrato, still a bit of the church choir treble in me, but it is a sweet sound. At the quarry though I sing alto, because my mum sings alto and I have borrowed her folder. Nice for a change to be hovering under the melody, I don't feel like soaring tonight. A fire is burning in a metal cage, smoke clinging to my jumper and keeping the midges at bay. Ash brushes my cheek and there is a bird somewhere making a racket but I can't see it amongst the rush of summer leaves.

Irregular Spanish staccatos ricochet around the clearing, and gently layered chords hover below the branches. Some of the singers have brought dogs, who lie obediently at their owners' feet. I take a photo of the scene for my mum, moved by the physical togetherness of real people as much as the music. I realise I have missed my choirs, the act of breathing in air and releasing sound on the breeze. It occurs to me now, wrapped in woodsmoke, that it might be time to rekindle my own singing group, reacquaint myself with whole faces, instead of only eyes. I file this thought somewhere in my mind as I follow my dad back to the car, pulling fragments of ash from my hair.

The next morning, we eat boiled eggs perched on stools around the table in my parents' little kitchen. Afterwards, The Mermaid clings to me as we load bags into the car and I have to unwrap her from my waist and hand her over to my mum.

The drive across to the Lake District from Weardale is in turn bleak, barren and beautiful, the landscape becoming greener the further west we drive. First we follow the River Wear into Upper Weardale, through Eastgate and

Westgate, then on to St John's Chapel and the wonder-
fully named Ireshopeburn, where I walked one day with
The Littlest One, counting sheep and exploring ancient
footpaths. There are so many '-hopes' in Weardale, deriv-
ing from an Anglo Saxon word and pronounced 'up':
Rookhope, Bollihope, Stanhope, Harehope, Killhope. The
name suggests a valley linked to a dale, ripples amongst
the hills, fissures that have been sliced into further by
miners extracting lead from the earth. The landscape is
stark, heather pushing its gnarly roots into the peat-rich
ground, hardy hawthorn trees slicing the air. In the twelfth
century, huge swathes of forests were cleared from this
area, as the feudal system gathered pace and a hunting
tradition developed, led by the Bishops of Durham. My
chest twinges when I try to imagine the lush world that
was hacked down and has never returned, the Middle
Ages massacre, a precursor to the deforestation that now
threatens our world.

Rising up through the dale, the road falls away on
scree-covered hills down to old mines, bricks from dilap-
idated buildings mingling with limestone rocks, layer
upon layer of history bearing weight on the banks of the
river. There's a lightness in the car as we climb higher, an
awareness that someone is missing, but also a sense of
freedom.

In typical fashion I am cutting it fine if we are to catch
the steamer at Patterdale that will take us across Ullswater
to Glenridding, so I'm driving fairly briskly while the girls
sing along to our holiday playlist. Through Nenthead,

where red squirrels dance in the Scots Pines next to the bridge, and on to Alston, the highest market town in England. The Mermaid likes to come to an organic shop here with my mum and buy herbal teas and rainbows of pulses. We are in Cumbria now and after a final vertiginous sweep up the road we arrive at Hartside, where the Eden Valley opens up far below us and the fells loom in the distance, silhouetted on this perfect summer day. Soon we have reached the outskirts of Penrith and on to Ullswater where the road meanders along the edge of the lake, dotted with people on paddle boards.

Patterdale is a seething mass of tourists. With only ten minutes to go until our steamer leaves I circle the dusty car park and squeeze into an almost-too-small space, then I get out and carefully open the back door so that the little ones don't smash it into the neighbouring car. Out they pour with fairy hair and long skinny legs as The Whirlwind bounces around from the passenger seat to meet us. I grab my rucksack and join the queue of people on the wooden pier at the edge of the lake. Across the picture-blue water, trees creep up towards fells dappled with scree and fringed with scarred rocks that lead to softly curved summits. We are quickly allowed to board and take our seats on slatted benches, shouting over the noise of the steamer and pointing at islands as we head north across the lake.

And time slows down, clock hands pulled back by an invisible force as we enter a world of Swallows and Amazons. Canoes row out to tiny islands, where children jump into the water or clamber over rocks. We follow with our eyes the path we will walk along to return to Patterdale, sometimes high above the lake, kissing the bottom of the fell, other times weaving between trees where cuckoos hide. We disembark at Howtown and walk up to a hotel, where we eat scones soaked in jam and cream and suck cold juice through straws before walking the five miles or so back to the car.

The world falls away, or maybe we fall into it, and the afternoon becomes a memory sprinkled with magic. I can recall dusty paths climbing up towards the sky, pointing out sheep to The Littlest One, who falls over early on and cries while I hold her tight and point at boats scudding across the lake to distract her. I can picture The Caulbearer running ahead like a tough little mountain goat, always freer in the open air, stroking bark on a tree or watching clouds form shapes high above her head. I smile at the thought of The Whirlwind in her Newcastle top and black jeans, a child on the edge of not being a child, and I wonder how many more of these days we will have before she has something better to do. I can see ferns curled like snail shells and boats curved into tiny bays. When I look back at photos from that afternoon my heart aches in my chest because it was such a beautiful day. And in the next breath I remember that someone wasn't there, that the reason this afternoon stood out was because I was able to walk for miles with my daughters, feel lost in a wilderness for several hours. And these daughters swallowed up the air, ran away the miles and this was what I had always wanted. But someone wasn't there, and what does that say about my wanting?

After ice creams in Patterdale we arrive back at the car and trundle up a track to our youth hostel, tucked into the base of Helvellyn. We are sharing a land pod, two double bunks stacked into a tiny canvas-topped wooden hut above a stream running from the fells down towards the lake. The sun is dropping behind the hills and I burn some logs in the fire bowl for heat and to deter midges. There are Pringles, grapes and some pizzas I have ordered from the kitchen. I tinker on my ukulele while the children go feral in the stream, shrieking and making weapons from sticks.

I am tired, lonely and a bit scared. I'm not good with creatures rustling in the dark: my OCD rears its head, and I want to be sitting here with someone making me laugh, adoring me. I try my best to be enough for my children, but at times like this I don't feel like I am enough for myself, and on top of that, I am missing The Mermaid. My family has already splintered into pieces, and the aftershocks are cleaving it further. I have visions of her making daisy chains, spinning under tree canopies and identifying birds I can barely see through the branches. I sometimes see versions of that child of nature when we are in the sea, I know she is still there amongst the waves.

The three younger girls are running around being tribal warriors, complete with peacock feathers stuffed into their ponytails. I keep catching flashes of a Newcastle top amongst the tree trunks and made-up songs about hunting are floating over the fence. A peacock is squawking on the roof of the youth hostel, and we sit on marbled rocks as the day fades, watching streaks of pink split the sky. Only six days and nights until the Mother's Moon disappears and I have not seen it since it was waxing. But now, we are sitting under a high ridge below the true heft of Helvellyn, and I imagine the moon to be hanging lazily on the other side, where I can't see it. I never find out though, and we must retreat to our double bunk beds and shut the world away.

In the morning I go into the building to use the WiFi so I can call The Mermaid. Two silvery men are sitting drinking coffee, all checked shirts and shower-smooth and not the usual youth hostel fayre at all.

Three of them! Are you all one family?, they hoot. Y*es, and there is another one at home, a fourth daughter,* I reply. *How marvellous! Four daughters!* And they continue to talk about us from across the room, about how blonde the girls are, so fair, and how can that be when the mother is so dark, they must have a blonde father. And part of me really wants these men to know that I was once blonde too, that the children are bursting with my genes, that I have poured everything into them, and anyway why do these men think it is ok to comment on what my daughters look like? I remember that The Mermaid has hair the colour of honey on toast and if she was here the silvery men would feel compelled to comment on it, like a thousand people have done before.

Last week, The Mermaid sat in the passenger seat of the car crying slow tears that rolled into her red lipstick until it smudged into the cleft of her chin. She told me she always feels different, and it took her a long time to tell me that, because part of her feeling different is due to her words sometimes struggling to keep up with her brain, and this means that when she is overwhelmed she can't speak. So I stroked the steering wheel and said *take your time, there is no rush, wait for the words to come when they are ready.* And as I waited, I wondered whether any of us feel that we fit in, or if everyone feels a bit 'other', and then I turned to look at her perfect face as she attempted to arrange her words inside her mouth and I realised that some of us feel more 'other' than others, and it made me want to try harder to understand her.

I find increasingly that I have to conceal certain bits of my life from people I meet. The difficult bits. The bits that are hard to hear and make the listener unsure how to respond. But the problem is that these bits are all true, and most of my life is wrapped up in them. It can start to feel as if I'm trying to create a more palatable version of myself, like a walking talking Instagram image.

On our second night in the pod, fresh from a swim in Ullswater and apple pie with a friend, we return to find neighbours. A London family. A friendly man, a calm woman and their two sons, a little older than my girls.

Fairly quickly the kids are all embroiled in a water fight while the London couple drink beer and I pour a glass of wine, and we decide to light the fire pit to stave off midges.

The inevitable unravelling of lives begins: *How long have you been here? Where do you live? What do you do?* and it is amongst this, as I try to be succinct, that I realise that my life is a stack of dominoes. As I attempt to explain one area of my life, I clumsily knock into another one. An absent daughter leads to Covid, then to hospitals and mental health, disastrous marriage and yearning for the city. By the time we reach Brexit I'm actually grateful that the current political state of the nation is almost as dramatic as my Eastenders life.

As my new friends throw bits of bark onto the flames and smoke swirls in the air, I hope that I have managed to convey a sense of impressive resilience, but it's possible I haven't. Usually, when I step outside my skin and hover over my family, I like what I see. I am proud of my life with my tribe of girls and I see myself more clearly now I have stepped out of the shadows. But next to these people, this unit that is firmly glued, each person's role clearly defined, my all-encompassing sprawl of mothering feels out of control and messy.

In the morning the woman hands me a receipt on which she has scrawled her mobile number. *Perhaps we can keep in touch* she says, smiling. *Do a house swap or something.* I am ridiculously delighted. It's possible most of my mess is on the inside.

* * *

I return to more appointments and more strangers asking me how many children I have and how I manage on my own. And the more horrified people are, the more surprised they are that one woman can keep this creaking show on the road, the more I wonder if the life I am living is impossible. Maybe I am not managing at all. Perhaps I am careering down a hill, picking up speed, moments away from a terrible crash.

I speak to a solicitor who describes my situation as '*precarious*', and I burst into tears with relief because she hears me and understands, but I also rather prove her point by crying and apologising profusely. She is not making a judgement on my life, she is simply saying what she sees, telling me that I am weaving gossamer threads that are intricate and delicate and likely to break at any moment if I am not extremely careful.

6
Flower Moon

Mead Moon, Horse Moon, Dyan Moon,
Rose Moon, Planting Moon

At last I have waved goodbye to the elusive Mother's Moon. Barely there in the sky but lurking somewhere amongst the waves. The metaphor of being slammed into the sand by a churning sea is not lost on me. This month I have been whipped up by a relentless, unseen force, and I imagine myself spinning in a whirlpool, desperately reaching my hands up for help while water fills my lungs. I have had barely any time to run, but it has felt as if I am on a treadmill, unable to slow down. I see my mania in the reflections of people's eyes, feel it in the skid of my tyres and in my racing heart.

One night after school I pick the little girls up from drama club. The headteacher tells me that The Littlest One has been sobbing. This is rare but I am not surprised, her world keeps shifting. Immediately I am worried and I am apologising. Blame and shame hover over my shoulders, holding me in a vice-like grip.

I turn to leave and my dancer friend is waiting to talk to me about The Mermaid, who she is teaching once more now that strength is returning to my daughter's legs. In the back of my mind I want to leave urgently because I have left The Mermaid at home and I can't be away from her for too long because what if she needs me? This is still quite new, this leaving her. And I'm thinking of The Littlest One in the hot car, wanting to check in with her and understand her sobs. But I stand and talk about The Mermaid's education, about how an authority has been in touch with the dancer and they are going to send a form. And she is so calm and gentle in her energy, my dancer friend, that she highlights my hamster wheel existence and I am drowning in words and apologies and justifications and diary dates and to be honest the whole conversation is a blur and I need to get in the car and be at home. Close the door and maybe never leave the house again.

But instead I drive home, spin through the door telling the kids to get into their swimming costumes, throw a lasagne in the oven and drive to the beach. Maybe the sea holds the answers. I park the car in a lay-by dotted with pot-holes, arguing with The Whirlwind as I struggle with bags of towels.

The air feels electric, not from any incoming storm, but from waves of panic and irritation bouncing around me. I feel like a cartoon character with lightning strikes flying out of my body and question marks circling my head. The spot I have driven to is wild and craggy, unlike the creamy beaches elsewhere on the Northumbrian coast. This means that there is usually no one else here because they are all looking for the grand gesture. I am so far beyond grand gestures today. I am a million heartbeats and fingers through hair and eyes brimming with tears, a cauldron of micro-gestures that are simmering and overflowing in a steaming froth. I lean back into the steep path, slip in the dust, and collapse onto a rock. As my breath slows and my head pounds I can hear intermittent cries, little screams. The Whirlwind has retreated, clambered to the furthest rock she can find and wrapped her long bunches around her neck. The Mermaid, who feels everything I feel, senses my madness and has disappeared into a shallow cove, floating in her happy place. The youngest two are dibbling about searching for crabs and dipping their toes in rock pools. I bury my head in my knees and want to break into a thousand pieces and be blown across the rippling water so no one can find me. So I don't have to look into anyone else's eyes and see pity or concern or alarm. The strange wails continue, and I glance up to see clouds of kittiwakes lining the cliffs. Hundreds of birds are wedged into the seams of the rock, darting out like dancers, their melancholy calls curling around me.

Across the cove, a woman rubs sun cream into her partner's back. I want to grab her adoring face and push it hard, tell her not to give too much of herself in case she gets lost in him. A nut-hard shell has formed around me, shielding something fragile and at risk of breaking, if it isn't already. Perhaps this is what it feels like to be broken, an eddy of shame and desperation whisked into a frenzy and hardening into brittle meringues that no one wants to eat. I wonder whether loathing is as contagious as the pandemic sweeping the world. Whether I have absorbed the mess of my marriage and converted it into a self-loathing that I am now seeing in the mirror of other people's gazes.

The Whirlwind has moved from her stand-off at the end of the rocks and is walking back towards me. I pull her onto my lap and she doesn't resist. I tell her I am sorry, and she cuddles me while a warm breeze blows her long hair into my mouth. I tell her I want to try to slow down, and this girl with the mind like lightning says quick as a flash *but not too much Mummy, it's good to be busy!* And I know what she means, she is so like me this one, with her thoughts exploding like fireworks and her inability to sit still. And I love that energy we share, knowing that it represents the very best of me until I am stretched too thin. I squeeze her tight, grateful that someone understands and loves me for all my faults.

The Littlest One has found a rock that she is cradling like a baby in her child-hands. They are still a little pudgy around the knuckles in a reminiscence of babyhood, but her fingers are lengthening which means I am closer to losing her. She has started collecting rocks everywhere we go. I wonder if she is trying to create a little world around her that stays firm and still, one where she knows exactly where everything will be and where she will not be surprised or confused. This stone is pretty ugly and I ask her why she has chosen it. *There is a mark on it here that looks like a lightning flash* she tells me. I watch her big blue eyes roaming the rock and want to crawl inside her head, completely inhabit her mind until I am only thinking about a mark on a stone. It goes into the bag with the towels.

The Caulbearer wants to stay, but somewhere there is a lasagne sizzling in an oven and we must rescue it. I tell her we will come back at the weekend to look for fossils and cook sausages. As we walk back towards the car I point out a seam of rock squashed inside some kind of Metholithic sandwich. The Caulbearer crouches down and strokes it softly with her forefinger, rubbing the dust with her thumb. The Mermaid points out a pink fossil embedded into a rock, and together we examine it as her hair drips salty water onto the sand.

Scattered everywhere amongst this mess of a day that I am desperate to salvage is mothering. These have not been my finest hours but they are all that I have. Later that evening as I sit in bed dosed up with antihistamines and paracetamol, feeling the effects of the vaccine injected into my arm that morning, I lean back on my pillow and watch the sky turn crimson. The Littlest One is sleeping on top of her duvet, mouth open, blonde hair splayed across the pillow. Next to me on my bed are three daughters looking for poems to read, singing silly words and giggling. My room is the smallest in the house but they have chosen to sit right on top of me, breathing my air and demanding cuddles. I hope when they look into my tired eyes it cancels out the self-loathing and replaces it with love.

The previous day, while the younger girls were at their dad's, The Mermaid and I drove to our favourite high tide spot, where glints of coal in the sand twinkled between my toes. I love to think about why this black dust ripples on our beaches. Over 350 million years ago, Britain was still part of a landmass in the Southern Hemisphere, warm swampy tropics and long limbed trees barely visible in the steamy air. Giant ferns and horsetail are embedded into the limestone, a throwback to the days when Scotland was attached to North America and England was still part of the European mainland. Millions of years of history dancing under my feet, streaming through my fingers. As I lie back on the still very chilly water, waves gently nudging me back to shore, it's good to feel insignificant.

The solstice comes and goes and The Caulbearer turns nine. The longest day of the year, although she was born in darkness, just before the clock struck midnight. She has requested a small party, only me and her sisters, and dazzles us in a blue sequinned jacket, sucking on a Sherbet Dip Dab. Instagram is full of #solsticeswims but I haven't had time today, and the days will start to shrink before I have a chance to dip my skin in salt.

After an evening of Musical Bumps and Pass The Parcel, the next morning the party is well and truly over. The Caulbearer wakes with a grudge in her bright blue eyes that refuses to shift. By the time we arrive at school she won't get out of the car and The Littlest One decides to make her own way in with an obliging teacher. I cuddle and I rock, and I think I am helping, though she will not tell me what is wrong, and I am not sure she even knows. Eventually, I slip her off my knee and out of the car, and she sidles into school, a mystery I cannot solve.

Back at home there's a packed lunch to make, hair to plait and a messy kitchen. Another one off to school and now medicine to administer along with orange juice in a blue and white mug, topped with boiling water. But there's the postman at the door with a parcel that has to be signed for, and he needs my initial. The cat is darting around the front door, refusing to come in, probably torturing a mouse. Meanwhile I have a missed call and a message and it is the out of school education adviser phoning to check up on me/see how she can support me to help The Mermaid with her learning. I call her back, apologise for missing the pre-arranged call and say the right things. Absorb it all so The Mermaid doesn't have to. Then I make a bagel and it is doughy and not what I wanted, so I make a coffee and that's better. I'm just starting to remember who I am when a legal secretary calls and I am submerged once more in the world of divorce and immediately forget what I was doing.

The morning continues like this and I have a sense of feeling slightly breathless, weepy in my throat but I'm not letting any tears out. I have one hour to myself this after-noon while The Mermaid does a movement session and I had planned to run. But the prospect of pounding hard, sun-dried grass in relentless heat does nothing for my mood. I am just too small today, too tired, and the irritating truth that I never feel worse after a run does nothing to guilt-trip me.

Instead, I find a podcast I have been meaning to listen to, drop The Mermaid off and drive slowly through coastal villages listening to a conversation on the politics of mothering. I sigh and peer over walls as I amble along, envying gardens sliced across with washing lines that swing in the warm breeze. The hedgerows are buzzing, the green of every paint-chart, and I'm reminded of early mornings when I would drive with a sleeping baby in the back of the car, horrified that the only way to get a moment's peace was to try desperately to stay awake whilst navigating country roads. Squeezing into hedgerows as tractors edged past me, brambles scratching the paintwork and a daughter behind me, head lolling, lips pursed and perfect.

The women on the podcast are talking about the need for mothers to find their tribe, and at this moment I feel like they are mine, that they are here in the car with me. Most of the members of my tribe are remote now. Moving to the far north of the country created plenty of distance, then my sister emigrating, one of my brothers setting up house on a mountain in northern Spain, friends finding jobs abroad, it all added to the isolation. And last of all the big one, the social no-no, the acrimonious marriage breakup, where different truths lead to awkwardness.

Soon after we split up, I felt a loyalty to my husband when I met mutual friends, swallowing down the horror, welling up when married couples exchanged soft glances or touched hands. I wanted that. I wanted to reminisce about student days and watch us all together with greying hair and faces drooping with age. Instead I held those friendships at arm's length. Maybe they withered in the breath of my reticence, my inability to communicate why everything was so very shattered. Perhaps the dynamics were all wrong, and the nights of dancing hard while he DJ'd and we pounded the floor together, sweating and smoking, laughing and dreaming, well perhaps none of it made any sense without him. A twisted truth and a broken past.

The global pandemic did a strange thing, cutting me and the girls off from the world. But during that time life opened up to me because everything was inside my laptop. I lived in the middle of nowhere but so did everyone else now. No benefits to a city dwelling when you are confined to the same four walls. And my tribe grew a little. I started to find people who sounded like me, wanted to engage with me, and it was the me who was just emerging from years of feeling broken and confused. Still the same me, but with space to try out something different. A suggestion of a shiny new me.

And so the podcast I am listening to, as I pass blood-red poppies in the hedgerows, crêpe paper flowers dripping wonder, has come from that tribe. I imagine for a moment that I have it just right, that I am not a full time carer, single mother of four, navigating a divorce, trying to stay afloat in a place that feels like an accidental home. Instead, I am the architect of my own destiny, gazing down on an oxbow lake that looks like a Thomas Cole painting.

The weather is hot. Properly hot, not Northumberland hot. The kids need sun cream on every morning, arriving at school greasy-faced and smelling of holidays. It hasn't rained here for several weeks, but Twitter threads weave stories of flooding in the south and a month's worth of rain in a day.

The Mermaid is well enough to be left with a dear friend for an hour or so and I run with my local harriers in the thick evening air, acknowledging somewhere this achievement, this escape, running so hard that my lungs hurt and it's nearly not fun. Except it is. It's glorious to be out, a pack of us whooping and chatting and laughing as a heron flies overhead and only I notice so it feels like it's flying just for me. There was a heron at the pond in the park where I used to walk with The Mermaid in South London when she was a toddler. She would run towards the railings calling *ari, ari,* for *heron, heron.* Years later I think she would still rather spend time with a heron than a human.

We kick dust up along the railway path, the world falling away beneath the bridge into a canopy of trees. Then it's up the hill where the air is stagnant, hanging heavy in the hedgerows. We sprint between the telegraph poles then walk, sprint and walk in a strange staccato pattern. The sea is a blue bandana ahead of us as we race down past the station, words strangled by the effort. And then it's back up again, through a stile and into a field partially mown and fringed with long grass, the sun still high above the copse. As we arrive at the riverbank, where I once saw a pair of kingfishers dancing under the viaduct, the temperature drops with my heart rate. One more push up from the stepping stones back onto the railway track. It's brutal, but I relish the physical intensity, the refreshing change it makes from the exhaustion of emotional onslaughts.

I arrive home wet with sweat, red faced and dead flies sticking to my skin. Yet The Mermaid comes straight to me, clings tightly to my waist and nuzzles her head in my shoulder. While my friend and The Whirlwind chat about football and I ask after the little ones, I know that The Mermaid is grounding herself. Rather like the cat performs her figure of eight around my legs each morning, to remind me that I am hers and she is mine, my daughter is remembering who she is. I know that even leaving her for these ninety minutes has taken so much of her strength. She will later tell me that she couldn't recognise her sister's voice, that she looked in the mirror and didn't know who was looking back at her. And I am quickly, sharply back in reality, in this world where I must always be alert, guarding my cubs from danger. And as my friend leaves, Percy Pigs scattered on the table, The Whirlwind crumbles as well, tired and upset. I walk up the stairs to check on my baby girls, and they are dozing in their bunk beds, waiting to be kissed and tucked in. Still smelling a little bit like holidays.

The Flower Moon is full tonight but hidden from view. Heat is steaming from roads pummelled by heavy rain, and the view from my window is a Victorian melodrama, flickering street lamps and raindrops splintering in the light. The absence of the moon brings with it a feeling of being unmoored, bobbing away from land. I can't understand why the sand is shifting under my feet when I know that somewhere behind the cloud there is a lunar orb gently holding me firm. Something about forgetting how to trust means that everything I hold is seaweed slipping through my fingers.

I miss the dark nights when I sat at my desk losing myself in the moon's gaze. This evening the sky is a listless grey smudge, sliced through with telegraph wires. A piano plays somewhere, bathed in luscious strings, as I search for a soundtrack that will remove me from reality, but the day is insistent and life is too urgent. Fairy lights dangle from my Grannie's bookcase, nailed on the wall above my head, and a candle flickers nearby, its flame stuttering in a pool of pink wax. The girls are all in bed, warm child-cheeks kissed, and if I make myself very small I can hold the moment and sink inside it for a little while.

It's Monday morning and I have another meeting on behalf of The Mermaid: another masked face at the door.

I had set my alarm early, but was woken five minutes before it went off by The Littlest One creeping in for a cuddle. Tucked her up in my duvet and ran a bath, in the process regrettably washing off my salty armour, still clinging to my skin after yesterday's swim. All the good intentions I had at 6am this morning are sliding down the back of the sofa and I am in every meeting I ever had where the walls are magnolia and the chairs look like they belong in a 1970s school staff room.

The visitor is talking while I flick through the pages of notes that have been written about my family. The words jump out at me like a snake's tongue, forked and venomous. I glance up, meet this woman's eyes, try to sense the kindness in the room but it feels drained and cold. I notice the spider plant's babies hanging timidly in the corner of my eye and crumbs on the table.

Endless times over the next couple of days I will be told that this is just the system, that this is how the system works. I wonder at what point I got caught up in this system, and whether anyone in charge of the system has ever had any need for help from the system, because it feels like the system is breaking me when I am sure the system is supposed to make things easier.

As I read the report I politely challenge statements that bear little resemblance to our lived experiences, and the woman politely challenges me back. I push as nicely as I can, as I have been conditioned to do, in a way that will not cause conflict or embarrassment, but slowly slowly she nudges me back into my place, squashed between the cushions on the sofa. The two of us are participating in some kind of passive-aggressive duel, protected (or confined) by a societal code I no longer wish to conform to. The woman believes she is doing what is best for The Mermaid and best for me. She is dogged in this belief. I continue to challenge and retreat, challenge and retreat, until one particular suggestion feels too much and I boil over. I don't shout, I don't invade her space, I don't threaten, I don't swear. I do none of those things. Instead I cry. Hot, sore tears that I try to trap in my throat but that spill out of my eyes and make talking hard. And these tears show this woman opposite me, with her knees neatly gripped together, that I am in need of support, that I am worn down by the demands of my personal situation, that I must be scrutinised further and visited regularly. But really these tears show that I am angry and frustrated and tired of unhelpful interventions and of being held to account for the actions of others. But I know which version she will be writing on her form and that silences my tears too late as I sink deeper into the cushions.

My body is as drained of energy as my living room is of warmth. The woman tells me once more that this is how the system works and the system knows best and I can tell she thinks that my pale face and hunched shoulders indicate that I have conceded defeat. She's wrong though. I want her out of my house so I can wrap myself in ribbons, burn bunches of sage and dance until my feet bleed.

* * *

Did you know that hysteria comes from the word for womb? asks The Mermaid the next day. I tell her yes I do know. Emotional, shrill and hysterical are the words woven into a false narrative designed to keep women in their place, when passionate, fierce and empathic are the truth.

I've promised the girls a return to the beach to make up for the chaotic lasagne-burning trip. The Caulbearer wants to find more fossils and The Mermaid wants to swim. The other two are just in it for the barbecued marshmallows, and it's an altogether different tribe that trips down the cliff path to the rocks today, hearts a little lighter.

The sea is steely, reflecting the sky which is bright and smattered with cirrus. The view from my rock seems to be layered up like mattresses on top of a pea for a princess - every shade of blue sandwiched together, fringed with harmless wisps of cloud. The tide is low, revealing glittering sand and shells that have been smashed into fragments. Predictably, The Littlest One begins to search for the biggest stones she can find and places them pointedly next to me. The Caulbearer, spindly and pale in her swimming costume, is dipping her toes into the water, white blonde hair falling in front of her face. The Mermaid is teasing The Whirlwind, challenging her to swim out into the cove towards the sea, knowing that this is where she trumps her sister with daring. The water is thick with bladderwrack and The Whirlwind has crouched on the edge of a barnacle-covered ridge, arms wrapped around her knees. She is fearless in many ways, so quick with her thoughts and words, but she is not a mermaid, she likes her home comforts. Her mind is similar to mine, racing ahead and imagining things that aren't there. Deep under the lulling ripples where The Mermaid lies on her back smiling up at the gulls, The Whirlwind imagines eels twisting around her ankles, crabs pinching her toes and a shark pulling her under.

I light the disposable barbecue, pulled from a dusty shelf in the allotment, and perch on some rocks with smoky hair and a shower of ash on my skin. Flames dance under the criss-cross metal and I start to spear marshmallows onto skewers. The Littlest One holds one over the heat, greedy to taste the sticky treat on her salty lips. Sausages quickly blacken as I try to turn them with sandy fingers and we pass a ketchup bottle between us to squirt onto clumsily ripped rolls. There is a thermos of tea - milky and a little bit sugary - and cartons of juice that spill when they are squeezed.

Kittiwakes shriek at us across the rocks as we huddle around the barbecue, crouching in towels that are wet at the edges where they have been dipped in rock pools. These are the moments that I hope will be stored inside my daughters' heads until they are old ladies. These are the moments I wrap up and gift to the girls as a token of a love that is wider than than the sea we are staring at. These are the moments.

7
Claiming Moon

Wyrt Moon, Herb Moon, Mead Moon,
Hay Moon

The sky is light when I wake and when I fall asleep each night, reminding me of the daylight hours I spent partying in Stockholm, stumbling out of clubs into a glaring sun that had never really dipped. We weren't married then and sometimes I followed him to Scandinavia where there was a decent demand for the bass-heavy Ghetto-Tech he played out in underground clubs. I used to find it hard to eat on these trips. Probably mainly due to a diet of vodka and cigarettes and my head not hitting the pillow until cafés were opening for breakfast, but also something to do with feeling unmoored, an insecurity that I couldn't place. I wasn't sure what my role was, apart from dancing in someone else's spotlight. It occurs to me now that I failed to define a role for myself away from him. Not for want of trying, I was singing, acting, teaching, throwing my energy into everything I loved. But somehow I was still being swallowed. I could stand on a stage in a packed club in Hoxton, singing blissed-out harmonies in a short black dress and cheap Hackney highlights and hands would be in the air. But I was never the headline act. Always the plus one.

The Claiming Moon is new and we are only days away from the long summer holidays. The school year has been ripped apart by various lockdowns. Structure and routine have felt very far away, but the pressure to be 'educating' has always been there in a formal sense, not in the holistic way I prefer. I am lucky that in the holidays I don't have to worry about childcare. I have made my work fit around my children out of necessity, because I don't earn enough to pay for much childcare and because there are only a couple of people I can leave The Mermaid with. This creates the obvious challenge of almost no respite, but it does mean I am not very reliant on others, so the holidays are ours to do with what we want.

The week before school breaks up we have a visitor. Anna is a new friend who has never been to stay in Northumberland before. I wonder how it will feel to build a friendship now, with someone who doesn't know how I became who I am. Whether she will notice a hole in my house where he used to be. Always I am working hard to show that I can be enough, trying to be two parents at once. I know there's a kind of arrogance to this - I can't replace a whole person and actually he is still around, just not here. Sometimes, though, his absence feels as big as the space he used to fill.

When Anna arrives there is a chicken roasting in the oven and we have set the table to make it look pretty. She arrives armed with gifts and the girls glow under her smile. We drink red wine and sit in the lounge after they go to bed. It's a novelty for me to have adult conversation, I'm used to falling into bed as soon as the girls are tucked up and I know I will be making a lot of coffee in the morning.

The next evening we are due to go out for a meal, but the skies are endless and my body craves wilderness not more wine. The babysitter arrives and we drive up out of the town towards the Cheviots. I want to welcome the new moon from the top of the world, with the sea spread wide beyond a patchwork of fields. It's about half an hour to my favourite hill, Yeavering Bell, on the edge of the Cheviots, a twin-peaked hill that is home to the largest Iron Age hillfort in the region. Yeavering Bell's eastern side is steeply sloped, covered in heather and dotted with wild goats that intrigue me. They were brought over to England in Neolithic times, originating from Western Asia, eventually replaced by sheep as favoured stock of upland farmers in the Middle Ages. The horns of the billy goats stretch to up to half a metre in length, curving behind their heads in ridged arcs. As we walk up a lane that edges the northern side of the hill, I strain my eyes to see their hairy coats that are often camouflaged against the heather, but we are rewarded only with sheep gently belching as a kestrel hangs high above us.

The incline is gentle at first, slowly rising out of the farmland until we reach a clearing, beyond which lies a forest. To the north we can see Scotland, an undulating spine of hills marking the border just a few miles away. A hawthorn tree and a huge rock sit just in front of a cattle grid. When I do this walk with the kids we always stop here and have a snack, and I take photos of the girls hanging out of the tree upside down and shouting *Mummy Mummy look at me!* It's a strange thing to have no one tugging at my hand or needing a wee, and rarer still to be able to walk without being hypervigilant about The Mermaid's responses to being outside.

I suppose she is a little like the moon, always orbiting me, magnetically linked. She would like never to leave our home, except to swim in the sea or visit her grandparents, and even those events can cause huge anxiety. If we are outside the house I become her home, the instantly recognisable thing that tells her she is safe. I know that I am blessed, but also that I bear huge responsibility. Most of the time I wear this responsibility like a cardigan shrugged around my shoulders, but occasionally it can feel like a loaded bag, leaving welts on my skin.

Anna and I are both wearing t-shirts and long-sleeved tops because the weather is mild, and a warm breeze strokes our faces as we gaze up at the mackerel sky. We turn to walk up a path that will join St. Cuthbert's Way for a kilometre or so, bringing us to the western side of the hill. St. Cuthbert's Way is a long-distance walk linking Melrose in the Scottish Borders, where St. Cuthbert started his religious life in 650AD, to Holy Island, his final resting place. I've walked small sections over the years, never yet joining them all up. The path continues on over Hedgehope Hill, but we must take a fork to the left that will bring us to the south-west edge of the base of Yeavering Bell. The path is almost completely submerged in heather and ferns that coil at the end like snails. The only indication that a path exists is a stone marker firmly wedged into the spongy grass.

As we walk, we talk about past loves and what it means to be women alone. There is something delicious about conversations like this, that unravel unselfconsciously. Between us we have both recently known great sadness, and there is an openness to our words that echoes the rawness of our hearts. At the very bottom of the hill a stream runs brown with peat, and the sky to the north billows like a fresh sheet. We walk up towards the Iron Age fort now, stopping occasionally to turn and look at the mist hovering over The Cheviot. Another kestrel hovers above us, and as we reach the crumbling ramparts, Northumberland opens up beneath us, a birds-eye view of the site of King Edwin's 7th century palace, now only a field like any other, but hiding unknown treasures.

We lean back against a crop of rocks and stare out at the sea, just visible on the horizon as the clouds turn pink under the setting sun. Jelly Babies and icy water feel like a meal worth savouring as a hazy glow settles over Yeavering Bell. The kestrel swings on thermals behind us and we begin the short but steep descent, an ankle-turning adventure on paths that are powder-dry from weeks of sun, especially in unsuitable trainers. The sun has dipped down by the time we reach the car, midges clinging to our faces and necks as we open doors quickly and sink back into our seats. This friend is both wise and open. I have allowed myself to be vulnerable in her presence, unwrapped some of my pain, and she has done the same. Funny how we can reveal so much of ourselves when we feel we have the permission to do so. Sometimes my voice might come out as whisper, but if you are willing to listen carefully, it can still be heard.

There is a gap in the endless restrictions and I have decided to drive to a campsite near Lochinver in the Scottish Highlands. Our car is packed full with a huge tent, blankets, books, games, food, swimsuits and camping stoves. The roof box lock is broken so I've smothered it in bungee cords and will have to hope pillows don't bounce out. I love the ritual of getting ready to go away on holiday with the children. Not the hideous dash to make sure I haven't forgotten anything, or the frenzied last minute wiping of surfaces and turning off of switches, but the little bag each child packs, full of books and games, a new magazine and a packet of sweets. When I was home educating them all, when they were tiny, we used to create 'Spotters', tick-box lists of things we might see on our journeys. They were scrawled in emerging handwriting that filled the page while an older sister drew a helpful image next to the words for those who couldn't yet read. And then the joy when we spotted a heron or a buzzard, The Littlest One always hoping to spot sheep and never being disappointed in Northumberland. There are no spotters today, just a car of excited girls. We wave goodbye to the cat, who will be spoiled by Elsie and fatter when we return, and head northbound on the A1.

Close to the top of the British Isles, we are driving along a road littered with passing places, edging forwards then being forced to reverse, two steps forward one step back. The road falls away down steep banks carpeted with ferns into lush green copses, where The Mermaid spots a stag only metres away. There are a few houses along the track, tatty and weather-worn, broken fences with splayed wood slicing the North Atlantic air.

The sky ahead looks lighter and I know we are close to the coastline. Everything is wider and whiter and glittering sand like ticker tape is scattered amongst the grass in the verges. Still no sea but a smattering of static caravans in sage and beige, and a sign painted in faded italics indicating our arrival at the campsite. We have been in the car for over seven hours, driven to Achmelvich, in the very north-west of Scotland. A tribe of girls escaping to somewhere even more on the edge of nowhere than our home.

I park the car on bumpy sand-grass and open the door. Washing is pegged to a line across the site, towels, wetsuits and swimming costumes being tugged away by powerful gusts of wind. A garage adjoins a tiny shop, which doubles as the reception and I stand in a socially distant queue behind another woman waiting to check in. The garage door is open, empty cardboard boxes and loo roll stacked in piles lean into each other. The girls tumble out of the car, legs wobbly as foals after hours on the road, and run past me to look for the beach.

It's been worth the drive. I watch them scamper through a kissing gate and down a path worn through the marram grass to where a crescent of shining sand lies waiting, tucked against a grassy bank. At the far end, the Highlands roll away beyond rocky crags wrapped in creamy lichen and dotted with orchids. And when I gaze over to the west I could be inside the pages of the book I finished last night, on the shores of a Greek island, because the sea is a big beautiful cliché, as blue as my daughters' eyes. My head is full of Hydra and decadence and I'm ready to be swept away.

A fierce wind is licking the site. It is blowing straight off The Minch, the stretch of water between the mainland and the Inner Hebrides, and across the field. We lay our 6-(wo)man tent out on the ground and the girls flit around trying to help. The Littlest One and The Caulbearer start to put poles together while I send The Mermaid and The Whirlwind off to find stones to bang in the pegs. The Whirlwind will do as little as possible, always hoping that someone else will do the job for her - brain that never stops but sloth-like when you need a hand. We are half way through inserting poles in holes and lifting the hoops into the air when a huge gust of wind snatches the tent from our hands and whips it across the field. I begin to run after it, then turn and look wildly for all of the girls. The Caulbearer or The Littlest One could easily have been lifted into the air, but they are running up to me laughing and shouting and pointing at our ruined holiday home, clinging onto my legs so that they stay anchored to the ground.

Putting up a massive tent with only small or disinterested children for support is a challenge, and my head is whirring with thoughts of how I am going to manage to pitch ours. Then, from all corners of the field, people come running, dropping what they are doing and racing to salvage my runaway tent. And all of a sudden I am apologising (why?) and grabbing tent pegs and wishing I knew which peg went where because someone who knows tents is asking me and I have no idea. But when I tell him I don't know, even though the wind is hurling us around and he has a holiday to be getting on with, he carries on calmly trying out different poles in different slots, sending someone for a hammer, making sure everything is properly done for me and for my children, and it is a revelation. I am waiting for the man to lose his temper, preparing to iron out the creases in the situation, save it with smiles and soothing words, but it's all ok, it's all just fine. Over the next few days the various saviours will nod at us as we pass on the way to the shower block. We are comrades. These strangers hammered us a home, pinned us to a patch of land at the top of our island, moored us on the edge of a cove drenched in seaweed, its rough edges framing the sea in a picture.

* * *

At teatime the sun appears, weak at first, a glowy circle behind the cloying cloud, but deceptive in its pallor because soon we have zipped back the tent doors and the girls are clambering up and down rocks like mountain goats. There is a strange brutalist castle hiding beyond the campsite, so we clamber over a stile and follow sheep paths to find it. The Caulbearer and The Whirlwind have whipped ahead, while The Mermaid sticks close to my side, barefoot as always, and The Littlest One is babbling in my ear about how Father Christmas manages to get presents to every child in the world (it involves a lot of elves).

The stone along this coastline is quite different from Northumberland, sedimentary stripes in vivid black and pink, like tigers we decide. The castle is very scary inside, *like a bear's cave* The Littlest One tells me, her eyes as wide as the moon. I snap pictures of the girls crawling on top of the weird structure but my heart is distracted by the sea, and the promise of a sunset.

The sun falls lower, casting a tangerine glow across the rippling water, sliced by occasional cormorants speeding between rocks. The sea feels bigger here, the horizon full of promise. I imagine Canada to be the next point of land as I stare into the distance, but of course the Hebrides are closer. The little ones are still climbing over rocks somewhere behind me, but The Mermaid cuddles right into me, needing an anchor to keep her safe in this strange new land, and tells me she is proud of me for bringing them. It's almost possible to forget the wheelchair that sat in our house for many months, clunky and hard to navigate in our skinny Victorian hallway. She is using her legs again and it feels so good up here, miles away from everything, the breeze gently tugging worries from my head so that they evaporate in the air.

Later in the evening we walk across the field to the crescent-shaped bay. The sand is as fine as caster sugar, and my daughters are dotted across the beach soaked in twilight. It's the stuff of dreams, and I wonder if I have found the place we will return to every year, the holiday where new, good, memories will be made.

The girls want the partition between the two bedrooms to be unzipped so that we are all sleeping in one long line. We take it in turns to inflate lilos with a foot pump and the girls unpack numerous teddies, books, sleeping bags, pillows, blankets and torches, quickly creating a cosy chamber. My bed is wedged between the two little ones, and on the first night The Caulbearer clings to me because the wind is still roaring and it does feel as if we might blow into the sea. I do my usual *don't worry, you're safe, Mama's here* line but secretly I wonder if the next gust might take us into the Minch. After a fitful night, light begins to seep through the green fabric of the tent and when I unzip the door the day is fresh but no longer angry.

I trial a new camping toaster, and it's a big event. The girls are laughing at my enthusiasm, exaggerating their enjoyment of breakfast with oohs and aahs and *well done Mummy this is delicious.* As I stack the bread on the wire frame of the toaster, crumbs drop into the heat and start to dance on the metal, hopping up and down like jumping beans, and I am suddenly transported to the house my husband and I rented when we first moved to the northeast. It had parquet floors and a long garden, and was part of my master plan to live the rural dream, a proper grown-up house for less than we had paid for our mouse-infested flat in South London. There was an Aga in the kitchen, and my husband soon discovered that if he dropped peppercorns onto the hot plates they would skip like circus fleas and create strange effects as he filmed them. I'm struggling to remember now why the peppercorns were so important, maybe we were collaborating on a music video, I liked to record songs while he created the visuals. It was one of the best things about us, the way we fed off each other's ideas. It was how we had started out, creating black box theatre productions for raucous audiences in a tiny theatre above a pub. My mind keeps coming back to those peppercorns, bouncing, and I can almost allow myself to remember what it was to love him, when our dreams still held real possibility. But not for long, because my eyes are prickling and I have to pull myself back into the now, where the hurt has already happened and I can file it safely away.

On the third morning the sun is burning the haar from the sea and the smell of baked seaweed is drifting into the tent. A haar is a sea fret, like the ones we encounter in Northumberland during the summer months, so we feel at home as the mist clears and the temperature slowly rises. I'm happily toasting bread while the girls drape themselves on camping chairs around the table, colouring in and calling out crossword clues. The tent smells strongly of nail varnish, there are tiny bottles of candy-coloured polish scattered over the table. I fish around in a reusable bag for The Mermaid's medication, snapping the tablet in two in another attempt to reduce them. Last time, a couple of months ago, the psychiatrist told me I could halve the medication, but within days I had lost her and ghostly figures hid in corners of the bedroom. We were falling back into a crisis so the meds were quickly upped and we had to accept that she was too poorly to manage without them. But I worry about the side effects, and know The Mermaid only puts up with the endless appetite, night sweats and hormonal changes because she is so poorly without them. Before this episode, she charted her cycle against the moon, measured her moods against the tides, but now Risperidone laughs in the face of all that.

Gently pushing the foil with my thumb, I hover inside a thought where I consider the compatibility of anti-psychotics with camping in the middle of nowhere. Hanging somewhere between horrified and exhilarated, the exhilaration wins as I add some Sertraline into the mix and lay the tablets on the table. Swap the Sertraline for Promethazine in the evening, more Risperidone after tea, but at least pain killers are rarely needed now for the aching muscles. Odd how ill health has quickly become the new normal at home but out of context, under the green glow of our tent, I feel brazen and reckless as vulnerability competes with danger. One moment The Mermaid is wrapped up inside her sleeping bag, the next she is swimming in a sea dotted with jellyfish. There is rarely a middle ground in our life.

But The Mermaid is gently unfurling. I booked this campsite with her in mind, hoping that between the sea and the knitted blankets inside the tent she would feel safe, and so far it has worked. This morning she will pull on a still-wet swimming costume, and when I watch her wade into the turquoise water the holiday is made for me, her recovery the biggest relief I could hope for.

Last night, as the sky turned pink, we walked along a footpath where cliffs fell away to rocks metres from our feet. Beyond the cotton grass lay a hidden cove, where we stripped and dipped our sleepy bodies in sparkling waves. A common scoter, jet-black against the fading light, swam in front of us with her two ducklings. The Littlest One jumped over waves in wet pants and a t-shirt, while The Mermaid clung to my waist. *I feel like I belong in the sea Mummy*, she breathed into me, and it was a fist-bump moment, memories of her flinching from invisible horrors, unable to move her legs, drifting away with the scoters. Back on the sand, The Whirlwind scratched at perfect sand with a spade and The Caulbearer stroked fragments of pearlescent shell, white hair blowing across her eyes.

*   *   *

Full of toast, and with fog lifting from the distinctive flat peak of Suilven, we climb into the car to drive north to a lighthouse where we hope we will spot a sea-eagle or a whale. Back and forth, back and forth, playing the passing place game in a kind of meditative trance as the holiday kicks in.

I'm aware of a colour wash of couples as I navigate this holiday with my four girls. Where are all the other single people? There's another mother on her own across from us with a teenage daughter and her friend, but they are a rare breed. Every time a camper van drives in off the NC500, there's a beard and a sun hat in the driver's seat and a long-haired woman on his left. Occasional lone wolves, greying men with cycling shorts who sit and read in the dying light pouring red wine into plastic cups. Young couples, tanned and tactile. Families camping for the first time with very young children, throwing crying babies to each other so they can hide in the tent for a quiet few moments. The type of couple I am supposed to be part of, with school-age children who still want to be seen with their parents, who are wondering if this will be the first time they have sex in three months. Couples with reluctant teenagers who slouch in the car over phones. Retired couples with freckled faces and weathered arms chatting over the washing up, reading and supping beer. Couples everywhere, but no one for me.

I almost don't care.

I am still in the act of retrieving myself from years of losing myself, learning who I am outside of a man's gaze. The Whirlwind finds an old playlist on my phone and Teenage Fanclub washes over me in nostalgic waves. This is his music, and for a while it was ours. But maybe now it's mine, dancing between the rocks and over the sheep that line the single-track road. *A crystal ball to see you in the morning.* Lying on a sofa in Holloway Road, hungover and a little bit stoned. Kitchen floor sticky with booze and whose turn is it to go to the shop for fags? No. It's still his song, but I can borrow it for today.

On the last night of our holiday I want to climb up high above the campsite and take a photo of Suilven, the mysterious protruding mountain lying just a few miles south-east from where we are staying in Achmelvich. I wander along the seaweed cove, tread carefully over wires trailing from caravans, past cars with windscreens draped with sandy towels and find a rickety stile jammed in the ground between some rusting strips of barbed wire. The little girls have come along for the ride, and as I turn back to look at the tent I can see The Whirlwind and The Mermaid shouting and waving at us to wait for them. And still I'm surprised to see The Mermaid running on legs that were aching and heavy only a couple of months ago. Occasionally I step outside of my daily routine to see what we have achieved and it feels like a miracle.

The Caulbearer, tiny and focused, has disappeared up the face of a rock. The Littlest One, fiercely determined, is following her sister, looking for the best cracks for small hands and feet. The older girls catch up and we scale the steep hill, emerging breathless on the top of a lunar landscape. A slim horizontal strip of cirrus cloud is stretching just below Suilven's peak, like a flying saucer hovering in the air. The rocks under our feet are fringed with mossy grass, the sky so blue and clear we can see right over to the Summer Isles. I am always scanning the waves for whales or dolphins, but the water is still, breakers occasionally flickering white and gently throwing up spray. To the north, the crescent beach is perfect, the turquoise waters we were swimming in only an hour earlier beginning in to take on a golden glow as the sun drops lower in the sky.

The girls are fearless here, bold and free. The Caulbearer in particular is attuned to the natural surroundings, needing nothing else for company except the moon jellyfish she spies from the shore, and the waxing almost-orb above her. We have needed this adventure after many months of being shut in a house drenched in illness and anxiety. For all of us there is a huge sense of achievement, of having found a way to holiday that works for us all, of having escaped and survived in this tiny pocket of wilderness on the edge of the world. The Mermaid is still as brittle as the shells collected in the blue plastic bucket outside our tent, but our life has grown to include the possibility of other worlds.

* * *

The dismantling of our holiday home is less dramatic than the pitching. I take a photo of The Caulbearer and The Littlest One wobbling around the field inside the tent's huge case like a headless alien and glance around me, breathing in the salty seaweed air. I want to inhale the essence of this magical place, know that I am holding it inside me until we can return.

On the long drive home, I shriek and swerve the car urgently towards the verge as a golden eagle soars above us. We are chattering, breathless, delighted by this prize, watching until it glides away into the valley below us. For a while afterwards, buzzards will seem puny, unable to match the vast wingspan and impressive beak of a bird we have been searching for all holiday. Like I say, I've always been one for grand gestures.

On the night of the full Claiming Moon I have invited some friends to swim with me and light a fire on the beach to celebrate my birthday in a few days' time. Birthdays are a funny thing when you are on your own. For the last few years I have celebrated mine mainly for my children, because they are excited for cake and presents. But I've forced myself to try to recognise my own value, used them as a marker for another year spent reclaiming myself. I have swum in the sea, imagining myself somehow growing stronger as the waves wash over me and the salt dries on my body.

This weekend the younger girls are with their dad. The Mermaid and I pack the boot up with blankets, logs and a bottle of champagne I have grabbed from the fridge. It has been there forever, waiting for a special occasion, and maybe this is it. The cyan sky is clear, arms bare in the balmy evening air and my heart is light.

The beach is still finely scattered with families and dogs. Somehow the sea has carved a crevice into the sand since I was last here, and beyond it the waves look feisty. The Mermaid builds a fire, and I collect logs from beneath the dunes as my friends gather. These are friends from different corners of my life, so they don't all know each other, but within minutes they have found a thread to hold onto, as if the sea wasn't enough. We are a gang. All of us carrying an ache that no one can see, relishing nights like this when responsibilities can trickle away.

The water is warm, surprisingly warm. But fierce. The Claiming Moon is nowhere to be seen but we feel it in the tides, dragging at our calves, pulling us away from the fire smoking in the distance. Over to the north-west the sun is a pot of molten gold, dripping into the sea and holding me in its glare. I am screaming and jumping and riding the waves with my arms held high above my head, bathed in glossy rays that make me shine. Further out, two of my friends, strangers until now, laugh and bob about, and I watch The Mermaid push through the breakers with painted lips and strands of purple hair around her face. The dancer is watching from the fire. All around me women are swimming and staring at the sun and the sky is burning.

After we have walked back up the beach, breathless and sated and dripping onto the sand, we congregate around the glowing logs and I pour champagne into coloured children's beakers. And we talk as the world turns pink, bats darting out of the dunes and moths flickering dangerously close to the flames.

Then someone turns to me and tells me how open and friendly my husband seemed last time she saw him. And suddenly it doesn't matter how warm the fire is because my blood has run cold and all the salt on my skin is not enough to save me. And I say to the friend *please can we not talk about him* and she says *you have come so far, done so well.* But it's too late. I'm back there again. Back to the reality of no one seeing what I see, and now on this beach with all these wonderful women around me and my mermaid daughter well enough to swim I am not enough. I swallow all this down though, put on a mask as effectively as my daughter, try to locate myself once more amongst the marram grass and the shells.

My friends hold me in their arms as we stand to leave, the sky now a gentle rosy glow behind us. Indigo clouds to the east. I could cry a thousand tears into the sand, drench it with my own inadequacy, but the warmth in my friends' eyes goes some way to stemming the flow and I hold them deep down inside me for another day.

The Mermaid hopes for a barn owl on the drive home. She is shaking and pale now, breathing laboured and legs giving way after the evening's efforts. She has ghosts in her eyes and I need to get her home. As we turn into our street she is tearful. Her head is full of horror and I don't know how to make things better. I can't even make myself better. I start rambling on about how great love inevitably leads to great pain, everything is worse late at night, all the platitudes in the world. And all the time the tears deep down inside me are churning and burning and frothing, desperate to pour out.

Later, The Mermaid has bathed, soaked away the sea-chill. I lift the reluctant cat, curled up snugly on The Littlest One's bed, and wonder if she is waiting for her to come home like me. The blind has not been let down and I can see stars glinting through smudged glass. I carry the cat downstairs and shut her in the kitchen for the night. As I go to check that the front door is locked, I decide to step outside and see what has happened to the Claiming Moon. Glancing down the street towards the allotments, the sky is an ink blot. A church bell is ringing on and on. It is midnight. Despite all these months of moon-watching, I can't pick a pattern out of the night sky. Realism crowded out by dreaming once more. The full moon is not where it is when there is ice on the ground, shining boldly through the window and onto my desk. It is closer to the horizon, despite the hour. Crossing over my street, I stand on tiptoe and look beyond my roof, where there is an orange glow. A few steps further and I'm flooded with something but what? A burnished Claiming Moon is full and real and right there, and I want to stand here bathed in her light before I cling to her edge and pull myself into her fire.

* * *

On my real birthday I am woken by whispers and bare feet pattering on wooden floorboards. Daughters pad through and bundle into arms that are a year older. The sky is subdued through my blind, but there are flowers on the windowsill, lilies I have picked from our allotment, and they are shining while the sun hides. In a beautiful coincidence, The Whirlwind has framed a painting she did at school of pink lilies and fashioned a bright yellow sunshine made from washi tape on the wrapping paper. And then there are moons: an embroidered one in denim on a card sewn by The Mermaid, and a scene fresh from our Scottish adventure from The Caulbearer, with a hare and a golden eagle posing beneath a night sky. The Littlest One has coloured in a cardboard mannequin to look like me - *you have had your hair cut mummy* - and written me a letter full of love. There are books and cards and candles and all sorts of treats from friends, and my phone keeps flashing up with messages from my sister on the other side of the world, my brother on his Spanish mountain top and my little brother in County Durham. The cat pounces over discarded envelopes and torn paper and jumps awkwardly onto the bed to sip water from my glass.

After a lazy morning we drive up into the hills. The air hangs thick and heavy around us, but the sun is nowhere to be seen. It's bright enough, though, as we pull up at the foot of Yeavering Bell and the kids tumble out of the car to hug my parents.

We've not seen them for over a month, and it has seemed like a lifetime to The Mermaid, who feels their absence like a caught breath. It's even warmer away from the coast and we kick dust up as we head along the lane towards the hill. Today we will only skirt the edge, pausing at the Climbing Tree for a coffee and a packet of crisps. We are walking to Hethpool Linn, a waterfall beyond the farm and the ferns, hidden below St Cuthbert's Way.

The Mermaid has a huge aversion to walks. For her, the only acceptable exercise is outdoor swimming. Once I brought her to another waterfall, Linhope Spout, tucked into the Breamish Valley. Standing beneath the roar of water, submerging herself in a pool surrounded by rocks, her face was calm, no darting eyes or jerking limbs, and I knew I was onto something.

Today I have double-bribed her with a day with her grandparents and a swim under a waterfall, and so far it is working. She walks barefoot, clutching my mother's hand while the younger two run ahead holding hands and The Whirlwind plays geography games with my dad. I can't remember the last time I walked for any distance with all of my children. In my head I have a very strong, raw memory of a day a few months ago when I was desperate to leave the house and all of its commodes and medication behind. I pushed my poorly daughter along the coastal path while her sisters slipped around her and helped me heave the wheelchair across the gravel. We were brave but fairly desperate, and when I look at photos from that day now I am full of pride but it feels like another family.

Those days of physical exhaustion and intense worry are buried somewhere inside me. Sometimes I am scared that I lock everything in a box, a compartment in my brain, just to enable me to function on a daily basis. The other day I took the girls to a dance workshop, and as we parked up on gravel that smelled of summer rain I saw parents sitting quietly in cars, waiting. I had got the time wrong and my children were late and I suddenly thought I would cry. My daughters were fine, they didn't care. My dancer friend smiled kindly, she didn't mind. But this tiny slip in the order of life had floored me. Another mum said something friendly to me and I murmured a reply, terrified I would crumble in front of her, disintegrate into the grass clippings.

But now the sun has finally risen above the cloud and my dad is forging a new path through a bog while The Whirlwind lists countries beginning with 'A'. I call out Azerbaijan and hear her cheer as The Mermaid leads us through the ferns and down into the gorge. My dad is slow and we wait for him to catch us up. He is a huge man, over two metres tall and so handsome with his aquiline nose and laughing eyes. He sits high on a pedestal for my daughters and they will not hear a word against him. His body is slowly becoming riddled with arthritis, but he is strong and stubborn, walking for miles through the pain. He is a man who has been defined for his whole life by his stature and strength, by his sporting ability, and sometimes I worry that aching joints and creaking bones will crush his spirit, but there is no sign of that yet. As we slide down the steep bank I can hear him telling The Whirlwind about the time he played at Wimbledon for his school, and she is in awe of her charismatic grandad.

The glory is soon over though, because he strips to his pants and wades up the river with a tree branch looking like a semi-naked St. Cuthbert, towards a pool where we all jump in. Dad takes the longest to submerge himself in the peaty water, shrieking at the cold and making his granddaughters howl with laughter.

We share a picnic of homemade tortilla and a salad of kale, broad beans and fresh mint from their garden. There's hot coffee and aniseed balls and really it couldn't be a better birthday. And the girls keep asking *Mummy is this your best birthday? It's a really good one isn't it Mummy?*

This is followed by another week of many appointments and, because none of the girls are at school, it's more of a juggle than usual. I'm trying to be slow, not rush, blowing out the stress and breathing in the scent of my lilies. By the end of one busy day, The Caulbearer has had enough. Her fairy hair hangs limp over her ears and her face is pink and angry. She slams her hand against her bedroom door and bangs it repeatedly as The Littlest One tries to get into the room to find her pyjamas. She's cross at teatime and folds herself onto my rocking chair, knocking it into the piano stool each time she pushes it forward. I try to winkle her worries out of her but she just says *I don't know I don't know I don't know* until I am almost tearful with frustration. Another daughter with no words and a head full of horror, I don't know either I don't know I don't know I don't know.

A while ago I bought her a notebook with a tiger on the cover. Some of the tiger's stripes are made from a purple velvety fabric that The Caulbearer likes to stroke. I had imagined that she might write me messages in this book when her words got lost. Today it takes an hour of very careful diplomacy and some advanced parenting skills to get to the stage where she is sitting on my bed writing a list in pencil. Because there are lots of little things making her worried she tells me. I wait for the list.

I wish someone would ask me to write my worries down in a tiger book and make them go away. My worries are endless. How will I manage when the children are on holiday with their dad after the year we have had? How will the children manage? Will the fallout be awful? I am not sleeping and I feel sick in my stomach. I am anticipating their absence and it is like a huge monster looming, a black hole in my heart. But it's Saturday night and the kids must eat, so I sit at the table with them and enjoy the domestic. I have roasted some vegetables, taken pleasure in making a rainbow in the baking tray, slicing red onions and fennel, watching the skin on the cherry tomatoes peel like smiles.

Despite the boom in women claiming to be their own best friends, lovers, their own everything, despite some women describing their marriages as some kind of purgatory, despite divorce occurring in almost half of all marriages, I still feel like an anomaly as I sit at my kitchen table trying to make myself a Friday night. The wine is bitter in my mouth, I know I won't sleep after a glass, and anyway the drink is laced with memories and regret. So despite the inevitable witching hour insomnia, I set an alarm for the morning and proceed with a day of running, swimming, allotment and cups of tea. All with four kids in tow. People smile when they see me with my tribe, and the single mother with four daughters feels like a better anomaly than the single woman.

The Claiming Moon wanes in a flood of tears. Rain explodes from the sky and within minutes there are rivers in the streets. Camellia petals are battered to the ground, a mush of peach and crimson, tiny boats for bugs. I leave the front door open because the cat is out on a prowl somewhere. Soon she will appear with raindrops hanging from her whiskers and fur spiked in peaks.

The sky trembles like a coal shuttle being tossed. The Littlest One clings to my waist as I watch for the lightning that must surely follow. A wet brushstroke against my leg and cries from a soggy cat. Dots of mud down the hallway and petrichor floating in the air. I close the door against the storm and wonder about the meaning of thunder in the middle of summer, why the world is shaken like a rattle when everything is steaming and you want to rest your cheek on a baked pavement and feel safe.

Maybe the Claiming Moon is a precursor to the dark winter days ahead. A reminder to remember the scent of skin gently cooking in the sun, know what it is to open the front door each morning and realise it is warmer outside than in.

The bank holiday weekend is drenched in a virus that soaks into my throat and lodges itself in my chest. I'm supposed to be running a 10-mile race across the middle of nowhere with my mum but my legs are lead and my soul is sinking. The kids are ill too and The Mermaid is floundering on reduced medication that has prompted the ghosts to return. I am spinning and flailing and sinking and how do I get out?

Next week the three younger children will go on holiday with their father for ten days and I am living with a constant hole in my stomach which I must get used to because it will not go away until the girls are home again, safe in my arms.

A not very small part of me thinks that this current bout of illness is linked to my divorce proceedings, which have taken centre stage this week. It's taken me almost a year to get my husband to sign the papers, and now he is actually signing them I can't really bear it. He is being interesting and funny and sweet and that was what I wanted but it's just the dregs at the bottom of the bottle the next morning. The hangover of a marriage that didn't make the distance.

8
Dispute Moon

Lynx Moon, Grain Moon, Corn Moon,
Lightning Moon

Somewhere along the way I have become fearful of dark nights. Sleep is elusive and blood pumps hard around my body as I lie waiting for grey light to filter through the blind. The Mermaid's bed creaks and I am convinced there is someone downstairs. A draft blows against the vase of roses on my windowsill and I catch my breath, or maybe I swallow the breeze. I long for a child to wake up and want me, distract me from the mess in my head, and simultaneously think how pathetic that is, how needy.

The days are getting shorter now and I thought I'd welcome the cloak of an inky night, but my anxiety about the children going away with their dad is manifesting itself as a grim insomnia and the darkness is no longer my friend. There is an odd contradiction between the nourishment I found in those winter mornings when light was found in candles and fading moons, and the edgy paranoia that accompanies these summer nights.

In the weeks leading up to their holiday I spend the evenings reading the girls stories, answering their questions, kissing The Littlest One's plump pink cheeks, massaging The Caulbearer's aching legs, plaiting The Whirlwind's hair. It's not clear whether I am trying to leave a little bit of me with them each time, like the scarf sprayed with my perfume I would give to The Mermaid as she screamed at the school gate. Or whether it's the other way round, and I am storing up the essence of my daughters like Rescue Remedy. The late summer sky deepens to a sunburn pink as I cling to these bedtime rituals and wonder who I will be when they are not here.

The Littlest One is weepy and confused and I spend a lot of time telling her how much fun she is going to have and swallowing down my own tears. It might seem melodramatic, this anxiety over a little holiday, but it is pain like I have never known handing my children over to a man who feels like a stranger, whose family have erased me from their lives. I am just a housekeeper now, the childminder, the one who made him homeless and broke all the societal rules, couldn't manage to put her husband first anymore. These are the people who will be caring for my children and I'm glad the younger three all have their dad's eyes, round and blue, so his family won't see me when they tuck my daughters in at night.

The Mermaid, who has my eyes, hazel and shaped like almonds, is staying with me. She stays in the car as I drop her sisters off with their suitcase and a sack full of teddies. I am working hard at being the good mother, waving the younger children off and trying not to squeeze them too hard one last time, but there is still a twinge as four become three once more.

I drive The Mermaid over to my parents' house, hoping for distraction and a long run through Weardale with my mum. I'm in training for the Great North Run and it's a rare day when I can get out and about for more than half an hour. The novelty of lockdown laps has worn thin, and there's something glorious about a linear route through the wilderness, and something even lovelier about being able to run with my mum.

Dad drops us off at Ireshopeburn, and we're over a stile and running along the banks of the River Wear as they pull away in search of a new swimming spot for The Mermaid. The sky is fairly dense with cloud, windows of blue visible on the horizon, but it's mild and we are in shorts and vests. Mum's clutching a water bottle and I've recklessly decided that I'll be fine without for ten miles. Always impatient.

I run ahead, occasionally circling back to find mum and chat for a while before I feel a burst of energy and sprint for a hundred metres. My heart is light despite the earlier goodbyes. Their absence will hit me in a couple of days, resurface as insomnia that leaves me nauseous and gasping for breath in the darkest hours. For now though I am running along single track roads while curlews trill up on the moors and the drystone walls pull me along a patchwork trail down the dale. Thistles are deceptively beautiful and alder trees almost perfectly triangular in the centre of sloping fields, hot sheep nibbling in their shade.

It's lush here in the summer, not southern lush where everything knows its place, but during these middle months the landscape sheds its harshness. It's easier to ignore the scarred land, torn of trees apart from hardy hawthorns, and lose yourself in the heather, purple as the smallest curve of a rainbow. And on the south side of the river the fields crawl up towards the sky, effortlessly dropping away before stretching across to Teesdale. Everything requires a little less effort in the summer. I only managed a few summers in these Durham Dales before I succumbed to a kind of winter claustrophobia and ran away to the sea, but when the sun is high I could run forever through these hills.

Back in my parents' garden I laze on a bench and rub lavender between my fingers, pull a flowering sprig of mint towards my nose and inhale. The Mermaid is happy here, tended to by loving grandparents who accept her for exactly who she is. I am endlessly grateful for the time they have spent reading articles and thinking about how best to meet her needs, and simultaneously resentful that I occasionally need to rely on them because no one else can look after my daughter. I'm bad at leaning on others, used to wearing my independence as a badge of pride, but the older I get the more I realise there is giving in the taking. Loved ones want to help, it's almost churlish not to allow it. It's possible that my reluctance to let others in is sometimes perceived as a door in the face, and without the help of my mum and dad I would only have half the life I have now.

In the evenings the four of us sit around a table and deal out cards for a game of Sevens, a version of Whist with a scoring system that requires concentration. We are a game-playing family, a passion that has been passed down through generations and is now firmly ensconced in my daughters, with the ultimate achievement being a win against their very competitive grandad.

I was brought up on games by my maternal grandmother, Gillian. She was widowed at little over fifty years old and my childhood memories of her are mainly of a single woman, my Grandpa featuring in only two of my memories before he died when I was three years old. It never occurred to me that Grannie might be lonely, though surely she felt my Grandpa's absence fiercely.

Grannie shared her home for a time with her mother, my great-Grannie, Irene, on the corner plot of a cul-de-sac of new houses in a Derbyshire village. She enjoyed growing vegetables - runner beans that we would eat with her homemade fish pie. I have the Royal Doulton dish that she baked the fish pie in, but now I fill it with allotment apples twisted from branches by my daughters' tiny hands, covered in crumbled, sugary flour and cooked until it caramelises. When I think of Grannie in her navy blue slacks and short sleeved shirt kneeling over the veg beds, I wonder how much of her heart she was pouring into the earth. Whether she was having conversations in her head with the husband she had loved and lost too soon, or contemplating the treatment she had for breast cancer not long after he died. Did she shake the soil from the potatoes, rub them smooth, wash them clean with the same care she used with my grandpa? Because all that love doesn't suddenly disintegrate - it has to go somewhere. Grannie was always caring; for her children, her husband, and then for her mum. But who was caring for her? When she placed her hands in the cool damp of the soil, I wonder if she felt small like I do, if her worries felt less in those moments, her place in the world assured and steady.

When we first moved to Yorkshire, Grannie would come and stay with us in our rambling old house on the corner. She would sleep in what we referred to as 'the twin room', which we used for bed and breakfast customers that my dad liked to call 'punters'. The twin room had a long sash window that overlooked the garden, a high ceiling and a basin in the corner. Below the window was a wooden seat which meant that you could perch on it and look out on roses that climbed the back wall of the garden and lavender that lined the path to the back gate, bees jostling in the air. My bedroom was on the second floor, so to find Grannie I had to tiptoe downstairs and try not to squeak the floorboards as I crept past my parents' bedroom.

She was awake early, and I always wanted to be the first one to see her in the morning. She would smile at me over her cup of tea as she sat up in bed with the shutters pulled back so the early morning light danced on the duvet. The advantage of being the first child down the stairs was grabbing the opportunity to tuck in right next to Grannie. My brothers and sister would have to climb in at the bottom and lean on their elbows, wriggling bare feet against me, but I could rest back onto the pillows, cuddle under her arm. There would always be games; alphabet games involving animals or birds; games where you had to change one letter to make a new word. Games I play now with my own children in my own bed, pillows stacked against the wall by my feet and teddies nudging my ribs. Perhaps word games fill the gap where a husband used to lie, distract from the memory of a hand placing a cup of tea next to the bedside or the caress of a shoulder through the duvet.

Tonight the ghost of my grandmother floats peacefully in my parents' living room as I sit at a precious table belonging to my other granny, crafted from walnut by her great-grandfather, a cabinet-maker in East London. The presence of the matriarchy feels strong in here tonight. My other granny, Mary, used to place her glass of ginger wine on this very table as she savoured each mouthful with gleeful enjoyment. Granny still drinks ginger wine every day, but the table came to my dad when she moved into a care home that can better support her, now that Alzheimer's holding her firmly in its grip. When I speak to her now I'm not sure she knows who I am. When I write to her I put a note on the back of the envelope for her carers explaining that I am Mary's granddaughter, Willie's oldest child, just in case it nudges something in her brain, pulls a picture from the shadows.

I imagine what it must be like for her when Dad drives for hours down to Devon to visit her. She is still tall and elegant, dressed in a classic knit with pearls at her throat, nails perfectly painted. She might glance down at her hands, dry as air, veins like rivers glowing beneath the skin, twist her sapphire ring round and round, the claw clinging to the stone as tightly as she grasps for clues. Sitting opposite her, the masked man's mouth is moving like a nightmare under black cloth, disfigured and grotesque. She will sip her drink, iced and sharp on her tongue, an old friend. Something about the man's eyes distracts her. She has seen them before, hazel and flecked with green, laughing at her. She remembers them dark and fierce, pupils like storm clouds, and again, gently closed, lashes resting on a freckled cheek.

Glasses clatter on a trolley behind her. The clinking and tinkling and scraping echoes inside her head until everything is bells ringing and a time long ago when the world was black and white, not this cocktail of colour and noise. The man laughs. Granny will stare, horrified, at the chasm where his mouth should be, fabric damp with his hot breath. His eyes though: slightly hooded with strong, greying brows. This is not a young man, although the way he is squashed into the ridiculously tiny chair, knees high to his chest, is almost childlike. And then the memory will appear, like mist floating off the early morning fields, a fragment of reality just beyond her grasp.

Trying to capture it is like taking home a cobweb in her pocket. Just as she finds it, it's gone, a tangled mess. But the spider is still there, weaving patterns out of nothing.

Back at home, I spend a lot of time on my back lane hanging out swimming costumes, wetsuits, towels and endless damp clothes. The sun fills this space for most of the day, burning into tarmac where the cat rolls in the dust.

Sometimes Elsie will open the garage door to let the heat in on her own washing and we will chat. I have to speak very loudly because she is quite deaf - when it is quiet in my house I can hear her phone ringing through the walls. The cat will rub against Elsie's legs, sniffing for the Dreamies that she gives her twice a day and Elsie will bend down slowly and rub the cat's ears.

Her garage is filled with tall piles of cardboard boxes. Sometimes on a Saturday, Elsie and her sisters, neat little Maggie and Doreen carrying her tiny dog, will drive to a coastal town a few miles south and park up on the quayside for the car boot sale. I have no idea where the boxes come from. They are full of Tupperware, teddies, tins, tea towels, maybe everything beginning with t. Except they also sell jigsaws, and every now and then I pop a pound coin onto a box in her garage in exchange for a new puzzle for The Mermaid.

One morning, Elsie tells me she must take Doreen to the local hospital because she has a bad chest. She discusses with me what time she will leave and the route she will take - *'maybe the coastal one because the A1 is so busy with the tourists, but if I get a tractor I'll wish I'd taken the main road'*. I ask her if Doreen has been offered help to give up smoking but Elsie says *no she won't stop smoking, she's tried*. That's when I notice Albert's grave surround in the garage, black and gleaming. I ask her if Albert used to smoke and Elsie says she remembers visiting Albert in hospital and taking him in four cans and a packet of fags to have on the ward. *Towards the end I had to wheel him out in his chair though*, she remembers. *He couldn't smoke on the ward then*.

The air around us on our little back lane seems to fall away and I don't know what to say to her, this woman who is telling me about her husband drinking beer in hospital while my cat weaves around his grave. For the briefest of moments, Elsie is lost inside her love for Albert once more. I agree with her that the coastal route is the safest option and hope that Doreen soon feels better.

Throughout my life, I have fallen prey to the 'witching hour', that bottomless pocket of time in the middle of the night. It must be a man who came up with the name, because witching is the very essence of wild feminine power, not a recipe for nightmares. Sometimes I become a sea witch, weaving spells in the waves, screeching and spinning in the surf. Witches are girls who rebel and dare to be different, women who refuse to conform, who challenge with their eyes. But the so-called witching hour still haunts me and is drenched in negative connotations of peril and fear. It rarely lasts for an hour, I know that from the blue glare of my phone. Time stretches, drapes me in its heavy cloak so that I am pinned to sheets that wrinkle and shift under my body. The squeak of a child turning in bed becomes a rat in the drawer of my bedside table. Night breeze knocking the blind against a vase is a stranger's whisper. The cat jumping onto the kitchen floor is a man at the bottom of the stairs waiting to steal my breath for good. There's not much I can do to break the spell – it is a trick of the darkness. Soaked in the night, I try to pour myself into a book, to lose myself in someone else's mind for a while. If the sky is clear, I can step out of my bedroom, heart bumping hard because of the man at the bottom of the stairs, and tiptoe onto the landing. If I am lucky there will be a moon, and this means I can breathe once more. The moon rejects the witching hour and spins magic in the tides, where the real witching takes place. I can bask in the glow splintered by my dusty window and wait for time to catch me up once more.

Sleep remains elusive. I manage an hour here, an hour there, but I can't really settle while the girls aren't here. Despite less physical demand for my mothering I am absolutely drained of energy, lethargic and removed from myself, almost robotic in the way I carry myself around the house. I'm eating less, not consciously, but it's possible I am trying to make myself smaller somehow, disappearing into a void until they come home.

Times like this a boyfriend could be handy, shake the woman back into herself and lose the mother. And as soon as that thought appears I give myself a talking to. Sometimes I'm bored of my own company though, the constant thoughts and ruminations, feel the need for something primal and physical. The smashing of sea against my thighs currently replaces urgent hands and perhaps for now that feels safer.

The nausea continues and I rub my gritty eyes as nights merge into days, and I am conscious of maintaining an air of everything being absolutely ok in front of The Mermaid. She sways between enjoying a quieter house and worrying about what is happening to her sisters. After they have gone away it takes a couple of days for her to feel comfortable inhabiting the house. She will start to feel agitated in the lead up to their return and then, despite being delighted to have them home again, she will need time to settle down once more. This is how life is for The Mermaid, a series of constant readjustments as she attempts to find some control in a messy world. She is acutely sensitive to everything around her, both on a sensory level and emotionally. I can feel her eyes on me, her body responding to my moods. If I am angry or frustrated I have to clearly let her know that I need some space for a moment, and later explain what I was struggling with so that she doesn't hold her initial response to my irritation inside her for days to come. I know that she will be picking up on my current state as an almost-person, as I drift between my head and reality, desperately trying to find purpose to my days.

When time alone is extremely finite it is difficult to know how best to use it. The temptation is there to work furiously to define myself professionally, separate myself from my mothering. But there is also a draining exhaustion that follows months of relentless caring, alongside the reality that I must restore myself because in a few days it will all start again. So my time is spent in a confused blend of reading and walking, writing and dreaming. Somehow I continue to try to write myself back onto the page.

One evening the little girls FaceTime me from their grandad's house in Dorset. Beaming faces burst through the screen and I gobble them down with my eyes. They are full of tales of a summer house in the garden and lemonade in the pub, swimming in the neighbour's pool and delicious pasta sauce. The Littlest One looks tired, crescent moon shadows curve under her eyes and I want more than anything to hold her tight, tuck her under her duvet and kiss her sweet cheek. The Whirlwind dominates the conversation as usual, relishing being the oldest for a while but also I wonder what effect her big sister's absence has on her, how she will carry this fragmentation around with her as she grows. All of a sudden she shouts *No! Come away from the window!* And my heart is lurching into my mouth as I see the shadowy figure of The Littlest One silhouetted by the sun. *Why is the window open?* I ask them, why is it open when there is a three-metre drop to the ground? And straight away The Whirlwind has her dad's back. *It's fine Mummy, we're fine.* And I know not to send any of my anxiety down the phone to them but it's there in the chills running down my arms, it's real. *I love you more than snails Mummy*, whispers The Caulbearer, looking up at me from under her eyelashes. And then I'm left staring at a black screen because they have gone, and I am sitting on the sofa with only the hole in my stomach for company.

After too many days of not eating or sleeping properly, finally it is the day when we will all be together again. It's strange how the world is a gaping chasm when my children are not with me, but when they return it's as if they never went away. I often regret the fact that the girls have to travel between me and their dad, wonder how that to-ing and fro-ing will affect them. Sometimes I resent him for moving to the city, for the journeys the girls must make when they could be playing or mucking around and not living with the consequences of our messy marriage. Other times I feel hugely relieved that there is distance between us. Mostly I feel grateful that I have been able to stay in this house with the girls, and as time passes I am learning to reframe our Northumbrian dream.

The Mermaid wants to make cakes for her little sisters' homecoming. It's still not a given that I can leave her on her own for any length of time, but she is engrossed in mixing and icing, sugar sprinkled all over the kitchen, and I will be less than two hours, so I swallow the worry and hop in the car.

As I drive down my husband's street I can see movement at the very end, a blonde head bouncing up and down in front of the the red brick terrace. It is my Whirlwind, and she is calling to her sisters *Mummy is here! Mummy is here!* Two more blonde heads dash out of the front door and straight away I am out of the car and they are in my arms and the hole in my stomach disappears.

Later on they are bathed and warm in clean pyjamas with small mouths covered in chocolate. The Mermaid is smiling in the rocking chair as her sisters fuss around her, pushing her backwards and forwards and giggling. She is the centre of their world and I potter around the kitchen, listening quietly as the girls call me *Daddy-sorry-Mummy*, but there's no need to be sorry, I'll be Mummy again soon enough.

One night I read some of Nikita Gill's poems to The Caulbearer, and I sit silently with her little head in the crook of my arm as I consider her words, *don't let a fairytale tell you who you are meant to be*. I had no idea who I wanted to be when I embarked on my fairytale. I'm pretty sure I no longer believe in fairytales, in the blind acceptance of happy endings. There's a danger in the belief that it will all be ok. I am still learning to lie alongside emotions that scare me: anger and jealousy and resentment are uncomfortable bedfellows. They are ugly feelings. But life is not always beautiful, unless by beautiful you mean raw.

* * *

There is something about the repetition of domestic life that lends itself to the observation of patterns: rows of socks folded over the clothes drier, spiralling pasta resting in jars, books on shelves leaning over like a sigh. And outside our home I am noticing the seasons changing, the way autumn is creeping in as bossy surprise, chasing summer out before it is ready to leave. Colours shift through the palette as the year ebbs and flows, creamy winter sun, brash oil seed rape, the muted gold of harvest and fierce orange sunrises. Hedgerows fatten with buds and birds, blossom and berries, then grow thinner, intricate silhouettes for the light to play with.

As the girls and I weave through our days, treading and retreading familiar paths, pressing our hearts firmly into the sand, pouring tears into the waves, I wonder if this is the power of the domestic. Tiny repetitive acts, running in circles around my back lane, walking up and down the stairs with baskets of laundry, pulling warm pyjamas over growing bodies, are these the bricks that build a life?

A friend tells me I'm living the middle aged stereotype to perfection with my sea witch behaviour, and as I amble down aisles at a garden centre admiring lupins I'm inclined to agree. But middle aged at least feels like I belong to me instead of following a man down a rabbit hole.

One evening I am pottering around in the kitchen and I hear a scratching in the wall in the adjoining dining room. Somewhere behind the drum kit and the Ikea storage filled with Lego and train track, a creature is moving. I desperately hope it is the cat until she patters into the kitchen and starts nibbling at biscuits in the bowl near my feet. The noise continues. There is a definite clawing sound, but also possibly a flapping, or is that my racing heart? The Whirlwind saunters into the kitchen and I pull her over towards the noise for support. I am no good with creatures moving inside my house that are not supposed to be there. *Oh I heard that yesterday* The Whirlwind tells me casually, as I imagine a family of rats making themselves at home on the other side of the wall. We had mice in this room a few years ago, when we replaced the carpet. The carpet has since been destroyed by the cat and I want to remove it and get the floorboards polished but I'm too scared that the mice will come back. And now I am scared that we might have rats in the walls. *It's fine mum* says The Whirlwind walking away, but I check very carefully for any gaps that a creature might crawl through before turning out the light and going upstairs.

My overactive imagination is a curse in situations like this, like a ghost scribbling images behind my eyes. That night I lie in bed and hope there are no holes big enough for the creatures lurking downstairs.

When I come down to make a cup of tea the next morning the cat is calm, curving her furry body around my legs as I pour boiling water onto the teabag. I am reassured by this - she is skittish and squeaky around mice, perhaps whatever it was in the wall has gone.

*   *   *

Later on, the children are all up in various states of undress luxuriating in the last week of the summer holiday, when I hear the noise again and my heart trips over. This time it is not a scratching. It is a frantic flapping. A bird must have fallen down our chimney, which is blocked off, plastered over and covered with a huge display about planets we made a couple of years ago. The flapping is loud and distressing to hear, amplified and echoey inside a sooty chamber.

I have no idea how to help the bird out of the chimney. I also do not want someone to knock a massive hole in my wall. I breathe slowly as I clear away breakfast plates and bowls and hope very much that the bird will find a way out on its own. I do not have the energy to rescue a bird today.

Two days later the flapping is still there. The terror that I feel at the noise in the wall is being nudged out by guilt that the bird has not escaped and that I have not resolved this situation. People kept telling me that the bird would die within a day or two and I tried to ignore it, but the flapping is still manic and I begin to think I am setting a very bad example to the children by not seeking a solution to the problem.

I google 'pest control' and find a man living nearby who sounds useful. When I ring him he tells me the bird is probably nearly dead and I end the conversation feeling defeated. The next morning though it is still alive so I send him a message and he is here within the hour. I can already imagine my neighbours wondering why there is a pest control van outside my house, it will be the biggest drama on the street this week.

The man at my door looks exactly as you might imagine a pest control expert in Northumberland to look. I am instantly reassured by an accent so strong I can barely understand it and his ancient flat cap. I feel certain that he will have tricks in the art of wooing animals that have been handed down to him through generations. This man is the bird whisperer.

I have moved a large box of Sylvanian Families and a basket full of handheld percussion instruments away from the noise. I explain to him that I am very scared of small creatures being inside my house and he must be extremely careful not to release anything he cannot easily catch. The man is looking at me with an amused expression on his face, and genuine terror trumps my annoyance at being completely reliant on this man and slotting neatly into a gender stereotype. I show him the back door, leave it wide open and scuttle out of the kitchen.

Within minutes the man is calling me back into the kitchen. He is cradling a small creamy bird. A pigeon. A racing pigeon, he tells me, showing me the tag on the poor bird's foot. Stepping onto my back lane he opens his hands and the pigeon rises into the air and beyond the rooftops in a heartbeat. I am so delighted that the bird is alive, so relieved I do not have a family of rats in my wall that I feel lighter than I have for days. I think this is the nicest man I have met in years and he is a 70-year old pest control worker. This is as good as it gets, and as the Dispute Moon wanes, it feels possible that this new lightness might be chasing out the dark.

9
Song Moon

*Wine Moon, Harvest Moon, Barley Moon,
Singing Moon*

Song Moon explodes into my life in early morning skies of crimson and violet, fringed with a crispness in the morning air that tells me autumn has arrived. I am rising early again now that the younger three girls are back at school, back into my routine of leaning my cheek against cool brick and watching a little grey tabby trot down the street. Somehow this is home, this ritual, and I am grateful to be hidden once more under burning skies, happy to trade the long days for a little seclusion.

My allotment paths are cluttered with sycamore leaves that curl in the afternoon heat. September is often a beautiful month in Northumberland. The sea is as warm is it will get, beaches are almost empty of tourists once more and the air is thick with the scent of harvest and sweet peas. I can hang my washing out on the back lane and it will be dry in no time, swinging between backyards and washing rooms while Elsie's sisters smoke and croon at the cat.

Mornings are earlier than usual this new school term. The Whirlwind has started high school and must be on a bus at 7am that will take her down to the city. The two of us build a little routine together that involves bag checking, hair brushing and cups of tea, and I feel so grateful that this fiery mind has found a school that will nurture her and keep her stimulated. She is my first baby in this sense because school's incompatibility with The Mermaid meant that rite of passage eluded me. The Whirlwind is almost a caricature of the preppy school girl, all bright eyes and bouncing pony tails, selfies of new friends popping up on her phone as she bobs in front of me with a hockey stick in her hand.

Once she's been waved off, The Littlest One will normally creep in clutching Lucker, her sucky blanket. We all have a love/hate relationship with Lucker (she couldn't say 'Sucker' when she was tiny and the name stuck). Lucker smells really bad, even though I wash him every few days. He is a small, dirty-pink blanket with a rabbit head, and The Littlest One still relies on him at bedtime. We love him because she loves him, but no one wants to be next to him at story time.

So in come Lucker and The Littlest One and we will cuddle on my bed before she reads her school book to me and that's already one job ticked off the list. Then the bunk beds across the hall will creak and that is The Caulbearer waking up and fastidiously tidying Mr Bunny into his daybed (made from a shoebox by the Mermaid). Mr Bunny is extremely elderly. Last year I had to perform delicate surgery on him, and since then he has needed extra care. He now spends his days perched in his daybed looking out across the rooftops beyond the back lane. He's enjoying a fairly relaxed retirement. The Caulbearer pops into my bed with sleepy eyes and maybe I'll read a couple more pages of something before it's time to get dressed.

I won't wake the Mermaid yet - she takes time to come round in the mornings. In a while I will take her up a hot orange juice with her morning medication, place an extra pillow behind her head and lift the blind. Her words might still be arranging themselves, the world still coming into focus, so I will stroke her legs, kiss her forehead and leave her to enter the day in her own time.

The school run is full of heron-spotting, bunny-searching and songs. Sometimes we have to wait at the level crossing and we will try to guess which way the train will come, left or right, while I glance at sparrows in the hedgerow and puffs of Himalayan Balsam float across the car.

Song Moon is still growing. The nights are cloudy and I only see the moon when I stand in the back bedroom to close the blind. The Caulbearer lies underneath her giant unicorn and The Littlest One is buried under a mound of sheep. Earlier today she read that people eat sheep and she cried on my knee. Now she is hidden under four fluffy sheep teddies, sucking Lucker, and outside there is a strange light glowing behind the chimney stack. The clouds are moving quickly across the sky and momentarily revealing the Song Moon as a milky jewel. Later on, when I am dipping in and out of sleep, I imagine it to be high above our house, whispering sweet lullabies that wrap themselves around my babies.

Last year as lockdown eased a little to allow exercise beyond our own front door, my children and I spent many hours hidden below the gorse bushes, on the rocks of Rumbling Kern.

Rumbling Kern is a tiny cove on the Northumbrian coast. In order to reach it, you walk down a grassy lane, past fields of pedigree cows, through a gateway caked in gorse. Beyond the yellow flowers, with their petals like kisses, lies the North Sea, stretching down beyond the fishing port of Amble in the south, and towards the Farne Islands in the north. If you shield your eyes from the glare and look directly east, it is easy to imagine Viking long-boats, shields glinting in the sun. On a grey day, when the waves crash hard into the rocks, dragging sand and tugging at seaweed, cuddy ducks shelter in the cove and the clouds fling themselves across the sky. This is where the land ends and the sea begins, a liminal zone criss-crossed by the tides.

Years ago, it was a haven for whisky smugglers, who would hide their goods amongst the rocks. Around the same time, in the early 19th century, Earl Grey built a bath house there to aid the home education of his fifteen children. Just below the house, two rock pools were created, accessed by steps carved into the stone.

The pool that had entertained Earl Grey's children became a focal point for my own girls, who squealed in the water and kept an eye out for pirates. I would build myself a little nest on the carved step and watch the oystercatchers playing in the surf. That summer we saw our first Northumbrian dolphins and a harbour porpoise gleaming in the waves.

As the children played, I would sometimes walk barefoot over the rocks, dotted with fossils, and sit just above the point where the sea threw spray into the warm, salty air. I would quietly sing the lyrics of Northumbrian folk songs I have grown to love: *Maa Bonny Lad* maybe, or *The Water of Tyne*. I would feel the years fall away, as if no time had passed at all and I was the first girl ever to sing those words.

I started recording little videos, holding my phone up to the sea, slowly scanning the waves, singing songs about loss and love and all those emotions humans have felt since they scratched their lives into the walls of caves. And the act of sitting on the edge of the world, as terns fell from the sky, and raising my voice, meant that I wasn't alone.

Over the course of that strange spring and summer, with our world narrowed and minds confused, I sang on old railway lines about ash groves and in woodland about blackbirds. On a particularly fierce stormy day, as the sky and the sea merged and the wind stole my breath, I raged through a version of *Blue Bleazin' Blind Drunk*, a raw folk song about the ravages of domestic violence. And one evening at Alnmouth beach, with the sea as still as treacle, I sang one of my own compositions, *Still*, as the sky turned pink and the sun dropped off the edge of the horizon.

These recordings became a meditation, a way of connecting with the world and, in a strange way, with other humans. As masks covered faces and people crossed the street to avoid airborne germs, the act of singing in the wild helped me to stay grounded and release emotions that were buried under the weight of a collective grief.

As summer leaked into autumn and a chill blew through the hedgerows, people tentatively began to meet at a distance and connect in person. I had felt the absence of harmonies keenly over those months: the process of layering my own vocals over and over on my phone was not as satisfying as the crunches and richness of other voices against my own. The previous year, I had set up a singing group for women. It grew from a place of need, a desire to be creative with other women, but it was also a way of giving something back, sharing my knowledge and creating a safe space. By necessity, I had to keep the number of singers down to ten: rehearsals would take place in my little living room while the girls slept or sang along upstairs. As the first lockdown came to an end it became clear we would need to find somewhere else to sing, a place where the air was fresh, because my living room had become a potential viral breeding ground and ceased to be safe.

Burnside is a tenanted farm in North Northumberland, a few miles inland from the coast, and a short drive into the market town of Alnwick. The land has been worked for years by my friend Linda and her family. One September morning, a trail of cars trundled up a long, bumpy lane scattered with pheasants, and parked outside her barn. Behind the farmhouse, a field stretched up towards a copse of pine trees, and sheep could be heard bleating in the distance. A group of women stood apart from each other, blinking at the novelty of new faces, eyes seeking out smiles that had been hidden for so long.

Linda opened the gate and I headed up the hill with these women, music stand under my arm, collie yapping around my feet. A buzzard circled overhead, high on the thermals, speckled underwings flashing. Over to the east, the sea was a slash of blue. Look the other way and The Cheviot erupted beyond the fields, shrouded in cloud. As we approached the top of the hill a huge hare ran out of the thistles, ears folded back against its head. The fresh autumn breeze whipped around us as we formed a circle, feet sunken in the earth.

The singers started wrapping their coats around them and donning hats, so we moved down behind the copse, where the air was still and sun warmed our faces. We discussed the lyrics of Welsh song *Migildi Magildi* as I strummed my ukulele - '*When the sea comes o'er the mountains*'. Voices floated gently over the fields and cows mooed in appreciation. The acoustics outside meant that I had to drop my voice to hear the soft harmonies of the women singing in a circle with me. These were women who work, look after children, care for parents or partners, women who quietly change lives, and came that day to sing in a field with me to care for themselves. By singing tunes that echoed through the years, we not only connected with each other, but also with the people who had shared the land before us. We became another thread in the story, our voices weaving through the hedgerows.

Long after we have gone, Rumbling Kern will hold the laughter of four little girls, just as the footsteps of smugglers lie hidden in the marram grass, and shadows of Earl Grey's children dance among the rock pools. My lockdown songs will be carried on the wings of sanderlings as they fly low over the sea, just a memory of a moment in time.

In the lounge The Mermaid is drifting between worlds, her eyes flickering and rolling back in a face that is pale and drawn. Over the summer she found a steady rhythm, her body and mind growing more resilient, but the return to a different routine and the looming shadow of formal education has triggered some difficult feelings. I phone her psychiatrist because she is in pain and I can no longer remember what is normal different and what is worrying different. The marker on her health spectrum over the last year has lurched alarmingly from crisis to crisis and I'm not sure what I'm expected to manage any more. Several times I have phoned for help when The Mermaid has told me she can't bear the anguish. She pulls at her eyelashes and scratches her arms. *Keep her safe* they say, *keep her safe*. And I wonder what else they think I am doing?

Keep her safe.

My life is keeping her safe, keeping them all safe. The words don't feel like advice or a solution they feel like a reminder, as if I might have forgotten what a mother is supposed to do.

Keep her safe.

So when the spasms start this evening, the jerking and the little moans as her beautiful eyes the colour of autumn fling backwards into the darkness of her mind, I tell myself to keep her safe.

Keep her safe.

And The Whirlwind chatters on in the kitchen to her as I phone the psychiatrist, because she knows the rule is Keep Her Safe, as if the grotesque twisting on her big sister's face is all just part of the plan. And the psychiatrist is not there, the duty doctors all go home at 5pm and *have you tried the GP and if not why not try 111?* And at that point I know I must just Keep Her Safe because 111 will tell me to go to A&E and I can't do that with four children in tow including one in isolation because of the global pandemic. So I put the phone down and I kneel on the floor as The Whirlwind creeps off to play with The Littlest One. And I stroke The Mermaid's tense little face, breathe in the smell of her hair. And I tell her she is safe. *Mummy is here and you are safe. I will Keep You Safe.* And I say it again and again until I start to believe it because what else is there?

* * *

Song Moon

A couple of nights before the moon is full, The Caulbearer cannot sleep. Her hot hand grips my fingers as I stroke her hair and whisper reassurances into her ear. I lift the blind sewn by my mum, a night-blue fabric with flamingoes and tigers dancing in lines, and the sky is bursting open. Clouds are illuminated like jigsaw pieces, scattered above the rooftops, and at the centre of the light show is an almost perfect orb, blurring at the edges as I squint and smile.

And just like that it's over. A link in an email. The click of a button. All of a sudden I'm no longer married.

My heart is still as broken as it was four years ago, but thudding with a dull ache now after the excruciating pain of the initial severing. A smashed vase stuck clumsily together with glue still oozing from the cracks. It's not so much that I miss the relationship, but that the impact it has had on me is still so close to the surface. I am easily shaken and I wonder if I will struggle to admit that I am divorced, with all its connotations. 'Divorced' tells everyone that you used to be part of something, that once you meant the world to someone. It reminds you that everything is fractured. The person who you lost yourself in, the person you banked your future on now looks at you with disdain and irritation. But sometimes you catch them glancing at you and is there a tenderness there or is it just the way the light catches his eyes? And you are thrown because you remember what was and what could, should have been. And you must deal with this harsh new reality because you have four beautiful babies, and somehow you must make this ok for them, swallow the guilt, even if your soul has shattered into a million pieces like shells crunched underfoot.

It's the night of the full Song Moon and I walk through the town with The Littlest One. It feels like a twister is coming - leaves scutter across the pavement and the telegraph wires are swinging up and down in the wind. The sky is cracked open with pink shafts of light and I scan the horizon for a moon. My daughter begs me to lift her onto a fence so she can wobble along it like a drunk tightrope walker. I hold her hand as she treads on the wood, worn with age, her blonde ponytail blowing away on the breeze. Everything is kissed with an amber glow.

It feels like something big is about to happen, the air is crackling and alive. Any moment now our house will spin up into the air and toss us over the Song Moon until we fall with a bump into a technicolour land.

Later the wind blows against the blind. Song Moon is blurred and low in the sky, barely above the rooftops on the back lane. I must wait until it's up above the clouds so I can breathe again and the glow between us can work its magic. The girls keep coming to tell me *Mummy look at the moon look at the moon!* They want me to see it because they know I'm obsessed. We all are.

*   *   *

It is now dark when I wake and dark before I go to sleep. I like it this way. My life is punctuated once more by the moon and the days no longer go on forever. The stark days of summer left me flailing, moored only by the tides pushing against my sand-submerged feet. Sun-kissed skin and a freckled nose, bared limbs and salty hair - all of this was small recompense for the desperate rollercoaster in my head. Not just skin bared to the world - it felt like everything had been torn back to reveal sinew and muscle that quivered in the heat, curled up and shrivelled as the sun burned hard.

It is a relief to be cocooned in red skies. Back to the cat curling her tail around my legs as I turn the key and open the front door on the world, begonias merging into tangerine flashes that light up the end of the street. And once more I lean. Lean against the sandstone porch, add the weight of my feet to everyone who has stood here before on a step in this market-town. Press my heels into the dip in the stone, as if by moulding myself into the very fabric of the building I am making it my home. Because everybody needs a home, wants somewhere to beckon them when they are far away. Specks of dust cling to my hair and the stone has chilled my feet - I will wear the house on my skin today, see if it stays with me.

One evening I come home from harriers - I've been pounding laps with other people tonight, mixing it up a bit. The cat has taken advantage of the fact that the lovely friend who babysits can't work out how to close our front door. I am sweat-drenched under the streetlights, hair sticking to a salty neck. I wander down towards the allotments at the end of the street and it all feels strangely familiar. The lane is dark, no lights down here, and I make sure to stand in the middle of the road where I can still cast a shadow.

Another woman has been murdered in the last few days. Snatched from the street and dumped in a park. Sabina Nessa. It feels important to state her name, to say it again and again. If only the repetition, the photos flashing up on social media, of a beautiful bright woman swallowing the world with her eyes, if only this was enough to bring her back. As it is, women across the country are exhausted as men appear on *Woman's Hour* talking about the importance of sticking to well-lit areas, letting people know where you are, walking in groups. Women reminisce about Reclaim The Night marches they attended forty years ago. I remember being taught self-defence as a little girl and thinking it was a bit of a joke at the time. But it wasn't a joke and it's not funny and women's voices are cracking and straining because what will it take to stop the killing? When can we take a break from constant hypervigilance and victim-blaming?

I call the cat's name, don't want to walk any further into the darkness, feel my heartbeat hammering in my ears like Sabina must have done, feel guilt as I catch my breath because it's still in my body. The cat shoots out of a wall covered in ivy. I turn and walk slowly back up the street under a sky thick with cloud, following her as she darts in and out of the cars and skips into the house.

The Littlest One has a birthday. Seven years I have loved this cartoon girl with a joke for everything and a collection of funny voices. She was born with the biggest heart and the most engaging, open smile. I look into her huge eyes and they reflect the world.

When I was carrying her, her dad and I were already being pulled apart. I couldn't reach him however hard I tried. I tried to plug the gap, stem the leak, but it just meant that when the dam burst, the damage was greater. Like the canals he used to dig in the sand when the girls were smaller, waddling in the waves with chubby legs and clutching plastic spades. As the tide came in the sides of the canal would become soaked and collapse in on themselves, and I would watch from where I was breastfeeding on a blanket as the water swallowed everything.

The Littlest One floated in on a tide of drugs into bright light and cold metal, in a birth far removed from her sisters'. Perhaps this was when I first started to lose control, my womb stretched beyond recognition, unable to hold my baby firmly in place so that I found myself on a trolley in a hospital far from home, my children being fed by someone else for days. She spun head down just before the planned C-section, so I opted to have my waters broken on a metal table surrounded by intrigued medical students, sucked on gas and air and tried to ignore the hook poking around inside me. I stumbled to a room on a corridor leaking amniotic fluid and waited for the oxytocin being pumped into my veins to take effect. After eleven hours I succumbed to some pain relief, and spun out completely. I remember the midwife saying *she's not used to drugs! Take it easy!* A few minutes later there she was, bush baby eyes and a pink body smeared in vernix. Another baby daughter.

Less than an hour later my husband had gone. Home to his mother and the three little girls wrapped up in bed. I lay awake all night long on a noisy ward, with a sleeping baby lying in a plastic cot instead of curling on my chest. The room was full of people, but I will never forget the distance I felt from my baby and the miles between me and my husband. I didn't know it was possible to physically feel a void, but that's what happened that night. And it was the only night she ever slept for more than an hour or two for a very long time, over a year, as I lay on the shifting sheets and a voice somewhere inside my exhausted head asked me what was going wrong.

A year later a paediatrician decided that what was going wrong was me, as I wept in his office. The Littlest One was picking up on my anxiety, that was the cause of her colic. It seemed strange to me then that all of my pacing up and down the house, the endless breastfeeding, the lonely nights caring for her, they were what was wrong. My best was not good enough. I wondered if he had heard me tell him that The Mermaid could not manage school, and that I was now home educating? Perhaps he didn't realise that I had two other daughters as well as the Littlest One and the Mermaid? Did he not hear me when I spoke at length about the challenges in my marriage? Or understand that my husband worked fifteen-hour days and I had no family living nearby? All of this seemed to fall on deaf ears, because it was me who was at fault, and me who needed to create more calm for this baby who only wanted to sup my milk and sleep in my arms but would not lie down alone. Not after that first night in the hospital.

Today the Littlest One has woken up bright and early, hoping to open a couple of birthday presents before the Whirlwind has to catch her school bus. Normally the girls are with me on their birthdays, but tonight she will be picked up from school by her dad and spend the weekend with him. As light starts to leak through the blind, the Littlest One's bounce starts to wear off. At first I hope it is the early start, the hour that has been lost to birthday excitement. But as she trots down the stairs for breakfast in her beach school clothes she dips her chin into her chest and clings to my leg. I peel her off and wrap her around my neck. She is hot and pink and her tears smudge into my cheek.

I keep my voice soft and sing-song, talk about all the treats she will have at her daddy's. Remind her that she hasn't seen him for such a long time and it will be so lovely to cuddle him and play party games. The Caulbearer is nibbling Weetabix at the kitchen table. Quiet and self-contained.

I have bought some pain-au-chocolats for a birthday treat and they burn my fingers as I reach into the the oven with The Littlest One hanging off my neck. The chocolate takes the edge off her sadness for a moment but she is soon back on my knee, snuffling into my shoulder and my words are only sugar-coating her reality. And my reality is that I never want to be without these girls, I want to breathe them in and lie underneath their giggling weight. But I also need to learn how to be me again, perhaps even for the first time. It hurts so much though to shed the mother and what if there is nothing underneath?

I am standing at Durham Station. Autumn is snapping hard at the heels of summer, and I don't need my jacket. The cathedral glints in the bright sunshine, a thousand windows catching the light. I'm a little breathless from all the racing about this morning, the emotions of four daughters, but also because I can nearly smell London, feel the grime on my skin. I am escaping for a whole day and a night, wondering who I will see when I look in the hotel mirror.

It is only days since the email popped up on my screen telling me

YOUR DIVORCE IS NOW COMPLETE

The end of my marriage is now complete. Something is over and yet it is complete. I thought we were complete, but then we were broken. Am I complete now? Or just a piece of something broken? Complete is a strange word, like I am being gifted this divorce. And maybe I need to reframe it so I can swallow the shame and sadness of something being irrevocably over.

I AM COMPLETE

I will keep saying this until it feels true.

I have not been on a train for over a year. This one is busy. I sit at a table with an older couple who have just been on a tour to the Shetlands. I am instantly full of questions, memories of remote Scotland behind my eyes, but they shrug and say it was ok, the weather wasn't bad, and then complain about the lack of hot drinks on the service. I make a quick note to disengage politely and stare out the window, scarcely able to believe I do not need to pull out a wet wipe or take a small child to the toilet for the third time in an hour.

The sun is burning dew off the grass as England rolls by, becoming softer and flatter and eventually more urban as we approach London. And my edges are rubbing off too. I am reinventing myself through the eyes of strangers, evolving into the person they see, feeling my own potential bubbling inside me.

The train slows as we pass Holloway Road. As I look up the road north towards Archway I remember nights in The Coronet sharing two burgers for a fiver. House parties where carpets were sticky and drugs were handed out like sweets. A girl with smudged mascara in the kitchen, singing Teardrop by Massive Attack after a really strong pill, the soundtrack to our coming of age. Everyone wearing moustaches and admiral hats in front of my trippy eyes. Was I complete then? Was I complete and then did I break? I look back now and see the outline of a woman waiting to be coloured in. So precious and young. So clueless. I want to take her hand and tell her she is enough, better than enough. She is the world. But she is not listening, too busy shielding her eyes from someone else's bright light and getting tripped up by her own shadow.

Humidity slaps me as I get off the train at Kings Cross and the air is alive. I am straight onto a tube and wrapped in the familiar warm smell as I sink into a seat with my book. I love the yellow metal poles, the horizontal adverts and people with music in their ears hopping on and off. I try to look like a local, wonder if I stick out as a tourist, and remember how the fast fast fast suits my natural rhythm, how hard I have to work to slow down to the Northumbrian pace of life.

I climb out at London Bridge and dip into Borough Market, where everyone is young and chatty, and the air is crowded with noise. Fruit stalls shine like kaleidoscopes, people spill onto the street drinking pints in the afternoon. I break out of the narrow streets, where the skies are wider above the Thames and it's like I've never been away. Cocktails with friends I met through a screen during lockdown and layers of motherhood falling away and revealing someone else. It's not that the mother conceals me completely, it's that the act of mothering is so consuming, so distracting that it's easy to forget who I am. I will never fully unravel the mother from the woman, that's not how it works, but these rare moments away from my children tip the scales a little, remind me that there is a bigger world out there. That's why it's so confusing when the missing never disappears, the hole in the stomach when you remember they are not there. The odd freedom that comes with two free hands and no one to swing.

The school run is changing. We shiver as we climb into the car each morning because the sun is growing distant, waiting to see my sister in Perth and leaving us with only a pale glow. I need to sweep my front path, where leaves have blown across the main road from the allotments and piled up behind the gate. The grass on my lawn is no longer growing at a rapid pace - maybe one or two more trims and then the lawnmower will hibernate until spring. I planted a honeysuckle in the summer and I'm impatient to see it grow, want to get past this boring stage of a few years straining for the trellis. Give me the curved cream petals and suggestive plump red curls and smack me in the face with your heavenly smell. Always the grand gestures.

Sometimes we play music in the car - *Put on a banger Mummy!* The Littlest One calls from the back, while The Caulbearer folds her hands in her lap and looks out of the window. I sing. We all sing. And we laugh, because we love this stolen fifteen minutes. *Can you spot the heron?* I call as we drive through the tunnel of beech trees and down towards the Lion Bridge. There is often one standing on top of the waterfall, beady eyes focused on the hurl of peaty water rushing over the edge. If the heron is there we are delighted. This will be a lucky day.

Then up and out of the town, and if you look south across the fields, beyond the A1, this is a view that can break your heart. *A traditional Northumbrian morning*, The Whirlwind used to declare, when she still shared this journey with us. And she was right. The sun is falling in the perfect place to catch dew or frost on the grass, and as the days grow shorter the sky is often infused with a rosy haze. On the school run with a beautiful song, sunshine filtering through the windscreen and two babies in the back, it is bittersweet and I inhale it all.

The fields have nearly all been harvested now. Farm vehicles lurk behind hedgerows and bales of straw lie piled up high on the stubbly ground. I try to hold tightly to the light creating a ghostly green glow through the leaves of trees, because in a few short weeks these trees will be silhouettes against a wintery sky. Leaves are already stacked up in the hedgerows like papers in an in-tray, and flutter down from overhanging branches onto the windscreen. The weather has been damper: welcome rain after another dry summer has darkened the wooden gates and the tarmac, and I seek out colour in rosehips and yellowing leaves.

One morning we are merrily driving out of the town and up into the farmland that lies between our home and the coast. I know these roads so well that I am always alert to any unusual shape or movement. On this day there is a bird on the verge, next to a pothole filled with rainwater and a dead rabbit. The hedgerows are many browns, glossy and almost empty of leaves, so this bird is well camouflaged with its speckled feathers. Its beak is bright though, and it's quite a big bird, ravenously ripping at the exposed rabbit flesh with its talons. As I drive past I realise it is a kestrel, squatting on the ground. We see kestrels all the time, hanging in the air with a flicker. Once I was running along a path above the beach and a kestrel flew out from the cliff. It was such a treat to see it from above, the rusty wings, after being accustomed to the creamy underside high in the sky.

The girls like to be punctual, a calm start to the day. Nonetheless, I do a three point turn in a muddy gateway and slowly edge back to the pothole. But there are cars behind me now and I steal a quick glimpse of the bird gnawing at the rabbit before I have to stop, pull in, let the cars past and turn around again, heading back towards the school. The kestrel has gone.

Once the girls are safely through the door, hand sanitiser squirted onto small chapped hands, I sink into the driver's seat and put on the radio. I love this drive home. It's one of the only times I can leave The Mermaid, because she is asleep and will not wake. Thankfully, and perhaps surprisingly, she sleeps well. Usually assisted by an antihistamine that slows her buzzing brain down sufficiently to let her relax. Nothing is perfect. Everything is very much not perfect. But this fifteen minute amble along quiet roads comes pretty close: The Cheviot, ominous beyond the level crossing, a barn with a triple curved roof, made from red corrugated iron and reminding me of American road trip movies, a gap in the hedge that holds a flash of the North Sea, glinting and steely in the waning autumn sunshine. And the radio on, an interview or a podcast that shifts my brain from mother to woman, or at least pushes the woman a little further into the foreground.

I round a corner where The Caulbearer always peeks out of the window for bunnies. The bunnies are all too cold and damp to hang around for us now, so we usually content ourselves with the heron on the bridge. As I near the pothole, there is a large outline crouching over the dead rabbit once more. The kestrel is back. I am excited because I don't think I have ever knowingly seen the same bird more than once. The kestrel looks up at me with fierce marble eyes as I slow down, then returns to ripping the rabbit. I wonder if I can take a photo of this bird to show the girls, and turn the car around, stopping it close to where the animated pecking is taking place. The kestrel stops. Looks up. For just a moment I am lost in its eyes, bewitched by the head on one side and intelligent stare. And then in two effortless flaps of the wings it has turned and gone, flown along the hedgerow and out of sight.

I am swooning from the encounter. Marvelling and shaking my head in disbelief at the brief exchange. I drive home to tell The Mermaid all about the kestrel, how just for a moment I looked into its eyes.

The day passes like so many others: I am a bee dancing from flower to flower, never fully committing to a task, barely scratching the surface. Yet somehow life is happening, and I am living it. The Whirlwind is settling in well at her new school, creating a world that is allowing her to try out who she wants to be. One morning, I drive her to catch her bus and she climbs out of the car. As I wave goodbye she is pointing up at and smiling at me with bright eyes. I glance up. The Song Moon is leaning back on the lightening sky. The Whirlwind grins at me and sprints onto the bus.

The Mermaid is always doing, creating, making, experimenting. We have been told in the past that this is not learning, but of course it is. She just won't take an exam in how to knit a beautiful toy cat called Magda, or create a birthday cake for her little sister that is topped with rice crispie sheep, or complete 1000-piece jigsaws in a couple of afternoons, or draw the most intricate sketches of the mocktails she is planing to make for us all at the weekend, or cook a butternut squash pasta so delicious she could sell it, or sit at her sewing machine and create stunning dresses for her dolls, or write a play script to be performed by her sisters at Grannie's birthday party, or read every book she can find on midwifery. None of this is learning. Except it is.

I have been conditioned to believe that this is not enough, in the same way that she has been conditioned to navigate life in a way that makes her ill. I sometimes feel inadequate and guilty when I see other teenagers walking to school or taking exams. I have to work hard to shift the boundaries and remember that it's ok to step outside the box. In a sense, we both need to do this, reject conformity. Her neurodivergence is not an illness, although society can make it feel otherwise. Her empathy and curious mind make the world a better place.

I leave The Mermaid engrossed in a cross-stitch and set off on the school run. The air is chilly, with the sun barely reaching our side of the street until it starts to fade for the night. The kestrel is not in its usual feeding spot, but to be honest there is not much rabbit left to attack. The Whirlwind told me once that the most common cause of death for kestrels is starvation, and I feel glad that this one has eaten a good meal.

There is a winding road with high hedgerows leading into the little village where the girls go to school. On one side, the ploughed fields run at a slight slope towards copses of evergreens that dot the horizon. Beyond that, the sea is rolled out like a carpet, the craggy outline of Dunstanburgh Castle just visible on the headland. To the west, the sky meets The Cheviot, and our little house is tucked into the hill just beyond the River Aln, dominated by an impressive castle. 'Coast and Castles' is why the tourists visit this edge of nowhere, but the longer I live here, the more the hills call my name.

Telegraph poles dot the edge of this road, the wires between them strung like washing lines, with pigeons and starlings clipped on neatly as they swing. Something is out of place, spoiling the smooth flow of poles, and I see almost at once that it is a kestrel. I am less than two miles from the pothole, and it seems entirely possible that this might be the one who looked me right in the eyes. I am giddy with this thought, feeling more in tune with the world around me than ever.

Which is why I am gutted when I return along this road with The Caulbearer and The Littlest One, who are chattering in the back about mince and dumplings for lunch. In the middle of the road, just beneath the pole where the kestrel had been perching only minutes earlier, there is a bloody mass of feathers. Brown, black and cream speckled feathers jut out of the pulp at odd angles. The bird is too destroyed to identify in a passing car, but I think the plumage and its size give it away. And all at once my heart is in my mouth and there are tears and I can't talk properly. The kestrel's fragility, strength and beauty have grabbed at my heart. I can't bear it, this poor broken bird, smashed into the tarmac by a careless driver. My chest is banging and I'm trying to fathom why I am so upset by a dead kestrel. Careless cruelty and an absence of kindness triggering something in my brain.

The school run feels like an allegory for life: everything is there. My children, the sea, stolen moments just for me, life and death. The next day, the cartilage and feathers have been squashed hard into the road. By the end of the week the bird has been taken by a tyre heading north, spinning round and round until it falls away or decays. Gone, just a memory, and I see no more kestrels under the Song Moon.

10
Blood Moon

Hunter's Moon, Seed Fall Moon,
Sanguine Moon, Pagan Blood Moon

The moon is only visible as a fingernail on a screen, sent to me from the other side of the world. I can't drag my bones onto the street to scan the skies. I am soaked in illness and the sky must wait.

The UK government has opened up the world once more. It's rarer now to see masks in shops, and friends stand talking in the aisles as germs swirl around their heads. The Prime Minister takes a flight to Spain, where he buries his head in the nearest sand dune as scientists glance worryingly at the daily figures. Fewer people are dying, he reasons, life must become normal again.

And true enough, it is unlikely I will die, though others will continue not to be so lucky. But on Thursday evening I test the Whirlwind so that her school will let her learn, and I do not feel lucky when two pink lines appears in the small square window. I have been feeling heavy and tired all day, and something told me to do a test as well. Two more pink lines. I gather the girls, trying to remain calm but feeling incredulous and manic.

The Mermaid, who spent nine days in hospital following her own infection with this virus, as well as five months in a wheelchair, stands on the landing looking understandably wary. One by one, I twirl swabs in tiny nostrils and wait. The Mermaid and The Littlest One are clear, but The Caulbearer is not, which means we will need to isolate for ten days. In single-parent households, when one goes down, everyone stays at home.

Yesterday evening I was running with harriers, a group of us panting and pounding, chasing down the night. A liquid sky swirled above us like ink poured in water, still fading to the west with bright stars above in the east. When I run in the darkness like this, in the company of others so I am not looking over my shoulder, I feel like I am shedding a skin, as light as air but strong and a little reckless. I race the streets around my home in a frenzy and return home spent, a woman edging into the foreground as the mother drops back, blurry and out of focus. Only for a moment, but it's enough to remind me who I am.

But today is another day, and the adrenaline now pumping around my body is nothing to do with hill reps or timed laps. I am not a stranger to this process, we've done it before, but this latest setback is coming on the tail of many months of challenge. Worse, I can feel anger bubbling inside me as I think about our immediate reality.

Hopefully I will not die, but I am the only adult in this house, this house with no big garden where children can play. I have no family nearby to help me, my oldest daughter is recovering from a huge mental health crisis and finds changes in routine distressing, my littlest ones need their friends, I need to work, I need to run to keep my brain in order, but already my brain is not in order, it is unravelling and I am spiralling down into a place that doesn't feel good. I am not going to die, but it certainly feels like something is dying.

Shaking off the existential horrors, I contact schools, book confirmation tests which are twenty miles away because we live in the middle of nowhere, email The Mermaid's therapist to move her session tomorrow online, boil pasta and throw it onto the table. I am sneezing, my nose is blocked, my head is stuffed and feverish and, while this domestic crisis is playing out, the Prime Minister is sitting beside a Mediterranean Sea glowing under a slick new moon, his head stuck in a sand dune.

The next morning the sky is cracked and flecked and I drink it in because I will only see it from my back lane for days to come. The sea is a thread of silver and I want to be in it, need to be able to swim through these winter months - illness broke that resolution last year and it mustn't do it again. For now I sigh, there will be no sea today. We drive down the A1 to a car park patrolled by people wearing high-vis vests and holding litter pickers, where I spend twenty long minutes unwrapping tests, swapping children over in seats so I can reach them, swabbing noses and throats, scanning barcodes and sanitising hands. Even the workers at the test centre can see that this is a lot. There is pity in their eyes as they look through the crack in the car window at my feverish face and I match it with a feverish stare.

Eventually we are home, with The Whirlwind logged onto her online learning and The Mermaid sewing furiously, the in out in out of the needle restoring some calm to her frazzled brain. The youngest girls are bouncy, though The Caulbearer's eyes are scaly and dry, swollen inside her pale face. I take them out onto the back lane, where the sky at least is wide between the rooftops and the sun is warm on our skin.

I am slow and feeble. Everything takes longer than usual. But I am determined to create a comfortable space for us all. I bring out a chair and the stool my grandpa made, beautifully carved legs and a woven seat. A blanket, a cup of tea, my sunglasses and a book. Water for the girls, chalks, skipping ropes and a hula hoop. Keys to unlock the bikes. I hang some washing on the line, not wanting to waste the warm weather, and watch the towels floating up towards the plane trails.

And actually it is quite pleasant here, amongst the bins and the dust. If I close my eyes I can only hear laughter and playing, and the sunshine is seeping into my skin as if I'm lying under a massive buttercup. For days I will try to recapture this magic, chalking on walls and organising running races when the lane is empty of neighbours, but the spell will eventually lose its charm.

A cast of unlikely characters dances through my dreams each night as I attempt to fend off this virus with sleep. A man I sometimes run with who perhaps would like to do more than that with me. My father, drunk and aggressive, a very dark version of himself. My ex-husband, before life got messy. All these men crawling across my pillow, whispering to me as I twist under the duvet on top of a sheet that is so cold it feels damp.

The Littlest One is full of beans but wants me to cuddle her all the time and I am torn between wanting her to catch my virus as soon as possible so that we can hurry up with the isolation and go away at half term, and feeling guilt that I might be infecting my child. The daily tests remind me of those nervy days when your period is almost due and you can't wait to find out if this is the month two lines will appear. There's the same tight feeling in the stomach as the liquid creeps slowly into the window, but the delight is reversed.

The Mermaid is scared, absorbing all of the emotions in the house, pushing herself to pop to the shop for milk, an act which can terrify her some days but she is desperate to help me, keep our little family afloat. In my distracted state I am vaguely grateful that she is robust enough to make these trips out of the house, memories of a child unable to be left in a room for more than a minute locked somewhere far back in my brain underneath the viral fog. The Whirlwind is frustrated, her busy brain desperate for social interaction with friends, but she is forced to make do with endless WhatsApp messages. She is not unwell but alert as a cat waiting to pounce, her energy fizzing off her like waves hitting a rock. The Caulbearer stands in doorways with her scaly eyes, a silent figure tiptoeing through the house in a tiger onesie. She is more subdued than usual, flopping on top of me as I lie feebly on the bed.

As the isolation unfolds, an endless queue of days that look the same, I wake up to skies that glow pink, muted through the frosted glass of my bathroom window. It is too chilly to stand on my doorstep in the the mornings, the cold stings my feet. One day the girls' headteacher arrives at the front door with a care package, a huge bag of soup, bread, chocolate, fruit and biscuits. I am mortified as I break down in tears, so grateful for the kindness of another woman who understand what it is to be ill and locked inside a house with four children. The tears turn hot and angry when The Littlest One finally succumbs to the virus and our isolation is extended by another week. I breathe fire down the phone to the man calling on behalf of the government to check we are following the rules. He tells me he understands how hard the situation is and I am so tired of being minimised again, sick of words that do nothing but nudge me back into my box, so triggered by not being listened to, by being controlled by people who do not take the time to put themselves in my position. Everything I am feeling after ten days of illness with no chance to run under the stars pours out of me like lava and I never hear from them again.

The drawn out malaise of these weeks is punctuated by acts of kindness that momentarily make my heart skip: a neighbour leaves logs for us to burn, one Saturday a friend drops off a newspaper so I can pretend it's a real weekend, there are many bouquets of flowers that sit in vases all around the house, a decent alternative to the hugs we can't receive. When the autumn sun shines I sit on a blanket on the back lane while the girls play with hula hoops, skipping ropes and bicycles like children from a Victorian novel, their hair shining white against the tarmac. One day an elderly woman I have never seen before walks slowly up the lane towards us, carefully placing her feet amongst the potholes, frail as she dips under my washing line. I warn the girls to keep far away, while she stands and watches them hula hooping for a few minutes. My heart slows down to match her gentle demeanour before she carries on up towards the road.

My bedside cabinet is covered in drugs that I dole out to myself and poorly children throughout the day. The girls crawl all over me, little elbows jabbing into skin that is sore to touch, everyone always in my tiny bedroom and no space to be ill. Whilst I lie back in the middle of a pile of daughters the sky puts on a show, biblical scenes for us to gaze at that make the girls pause and rest for a moment. There is no moon for us while the virus works its way through my family, I am too tired to chase it and each evening the night comes in on a flood of cloud.

I wonder if the seasons will have shifted beyond recognition next time I leave the house, if the hedgerows will be bare and the sun hanging lower in the sky? Maybe the geese will have flown without me and what about the leaves? Will they be trodden into the fields or are a few bright yellow flecks waiting for me to wave them off for another year?

I wake up while it is still dark, the days shortening and light taking longer to creep under the blind. Lying in the gloom, I can hear The Mermaid's bed creaking as she turns over, a cough somewhere, and outside a car door banging as workers start to head out for the day. When I turn on the fairy lights that wind around my bed they fizz and bleed into the darkness like sparklers, illuminating a face starved of something. Sunlight probably, or adult interaction.

My body no longer feels feverish, racked with pain. Four nights ago I lay on the sofa and wished so badly I was in my bed that I told The Whirlwind I felt like I was going to die. Her eyes widened as I hastily reassured her I was being dramatic. I did feel really poorly though. I just forgot I was supposed to hold that inside me, continue to chivvy children up to the bathroom to brush teeth, cuddle them closely against skin that hurt to be touched, wipe wet eyes and stroke sore heads.

But now I feel drenched in some kind of viral malaise. Heavy, with a stuffed head and senses that don't work properly. I sit at my desk and light my candles, watch the flames flickering against my breath, but there is no scent. A cup of tea is warm on my tongue, but tasteless. I brush my hand against my neck, pull at the skin to remind myself I still exist. Turn my head towards dark grey clouds that are shifting to reveal little pink explosions. My world is getting smaller each day, shrinking as I try to dredge up more energy from nowhere to pour into children who are tired of their wings being clipped.

The Blood Moon is nowhere to be seen. One illegal night I tiptoe out of my house, pad in my socks across the road and gaze up into the sky. I'm grateful for cold evening air on my skin, a change in scene. There is no one around, neighbours all tucked behind curtains. I scan the black for a fingernail, a connection, something, but not even a star. My hands are wrapping a blanket around my neck and I am sighing deeply when I hear a noise. At first I think it is chickens over in the allotments, a kind of chuckling gobbling sound. Instinctively I glance over in that direction, keep listening, but the sound is coming from high above. My neck is stiff and sore as I tip my head right back and strain my eyes into the darkness. The noise is clearer now, almost overhead. Geese.

I have missed the geese. Usually the school run at this time of year is punctuated by arrows of geese slicing the sky. They make me feel more grounded every year that I see them. Pink-footed geese from Iceland, Brent geese and Barnacle geese flying south from the Arctic, where they breed. Thousands of them heading towards Lindisfarne Nature Reserve each winter while I welcome them back like old friends. The recent absence of school runs has denied me these encounters, but tonight they are back, high above my rooftop. The night is so quiet I imagine I can hear their wings brushing against the air. And somewhere out there is a moon, leaning back into the night, calm and constant, weaving magic into the tides. And I have to remember that one day soon I will be cloaked in icy water. I only hope I will be able to taste the salt on my tongue.

Slowly the virus soaks away, although I can still feel it in the dredging of my bones around the house and the dulling of my senses as I cook up garlic that smells of empty promises. I have stopped trying to engage the little two with virtual learning, we are eighteen months into this strange new world and all they want is to dress up in my scarves and inhabit different worlds where they are free to go wherever they want.

As night falls I step outside the house onto the street with The Caulbearer barefoot in a her tiger onesie. I lift her up and she wraps her legs around my waist. The cool air nips at my skin and there's no scent to the breeze but the atmosphere is alive and full of expectation. I start talking to her, telling her it has been so hard these last two weeks and she squeezes me a little tighter. She is featherlight, this one, but even so her weight pushes my hips out and my legs are heavy. There is something delicious about the gleam of wet tarmac and reflections of street lamps melting into pavements that fills me up as we gaze above the rooftops and are swallowed by the sky.

Somewhere out there the Blood Moon is hovering amongst the clouds. As it rises we will catch glimpses of a luminous almost-orb, like a winking eye. The moon is bolder now, taking courage as it grows, pushing through the night smudge, and we cling to it. We have needed it so badly with nowhere else to turn, no place we can run. We can only soak ourselves in its glow as it rises to the occasion. As bare feet patter across the landing and tiny pearl teeth are brushed I will be called from wherever I am, stacking the dishwasher or folding clothes, filling hot water bottles or looking for medication. *Mummy come quick!* And every time I do come quick. I run up the stairs where I know there will be a cluster of jiggling girls standing on tiptoe and staring up at the Blood Moon.

It is day 15 of isolation and with two days to go The Littlest One is almost broken by this extended confinement. She is weepy and fractious and I can't bear to look at her face through the car window as I walk The Caulbearer into school. She has suffered the most by being forced to stay at home because the rest of us were contagious and now she has to do her own time. The impact of government decisions on families that look a little different has been harshly ignored, and despite a fear of authority that sickens me, I take the long route home and park in a lay-by next to a hidden beach.

The sun is low above a treacle sea, watery through clouds creating a monochrome effect against the black rocks. We slip and slide down a path etched into the steep bank by curious walkers, holding on to strands of grass because our trainers are inadequate in the mud. There is a curlew calling and dancing along the shoreline. We decide to climb across the seaweed below the cliffs, all eyes on the horizon we have missed and the sea slapping relentlessly against the rocks. The Littlest One has cheeks that are shiny pink and she is pulling me over greasy bladderwrack, searching for safe places to place her feet. The waves are persistent, the tide hungrily clawing at age-old clefts and ridges as kittiwakes shriek overhead.

We steal fifteen minutes of illegal fresh air, hold hands and stare out at forever, before jumping over barnacles and reluctantly climbing back up to the car. As I start the engine I turn to look at my youngest daughter and notice that her body has lost some of its tension, her face is no longer pinched. The sea has worked its magic.

After seventeen long days of isolation we are no longer deemed a risk to society. We have served our time and The Littlest One leaps out of bed on a Sunday morning and throws herself onto me. *It is Freedom Day Mama* she breathes into my neck, and her cheeks are flushed with excitement. Today we will pack clothes and teddies into suitcases, games and books into bags and even our cat into her basket, and we will drive across the border to a seaside town just south of Edinburgh. I have booked us a cottage that opens out onto the beach, all tongue and groove and scuffed wooden floors. There will be jigsaws and stories, mussel shells lying in buckets by the back door, sea-drenched leggings hanging from radiators and little paper bags filled with old fashioned sweets that we buy from a shop called Sugar Mountain.

My parents will join us later in the week and I want to leave the children with them and run for miles along the coast. But I can still feel the virus lingering inside me and it has other plans. It feels inevitable that my body might not be able to fight back in the way I want it to. I have spent the last few years battling emotional trauma, grieving the loss of a marriage, fighting authorities, caring for a chronically ill child and mothering four girls. I have also been trying to create a life that holds meaning just for me - running, teaching, swimming, singing, writing - a life beyond my children. I feel that I deserve this, but I also know it comes at a cost. I think back to the flu I had several years ago, lying in bed knitting a black scarf, and I know that the physical ruin I feel now is a manifestation of all the emotional weight I have been carrying. I understand, deep down, that I must look for ways to be kinder to myself, though right now I am not sure how to do that, how to reduce my workload without shrinking my life.

One day in the pretty cottage on the beach it is mild. The air still feels like early autumn, though the mornings are getting darker and any moment now the clocks will go back and temperatures will drop. I am feeling a little brighter, the viral cloak seems lighter today and I want to be in the sea. I step out of the house with the girls, through the patch of garden with its powder blue gate and onto the marram grass that edges the beach. The Caulbearer runs across the pink rocks towards the shoreline, pausing to look out over the Firth of Forth, enjoying the sensation of standing in a liminal zone. The Littlest One is collecting sea glass to add to the dusty jars on a windowsill outside our kitchen: mosaics of green, blue and milky white collected with tiny fingers.

As we walk along the beach, the coastline to the south opens up before us, Bass Rock a sleeping sea monster in the steely blue as the children race ahead of me in wetsuits. Yesterday I found a perfect swimming spot at the end of the beach before it rounds the corner, but today the tide is too low so I must think again. We find a cave in this hidden bay and The Caulbearer creeps inside while The Whirlwind finds writing engraved upon a nearby rock and begins to concoct a deadly tale involving intrigue and murder. There is grass between the rocks on this stretch of coast, cream and mustard lichen clinging to them as I sit down on one and look down at the beach where The Littlest One is still gathering treasure. Words from a spooky story float from the cave and mingle in the rockpools.

When we walk back towards the cottage I am still looking out for somewhere deep enough to swim that is not drenched in seaweed. There is no way The Whirlwind is coming in, she's perching on a rock in smart trainers and a denim jacket, but the little two are hovering on the shoreline in their wetsuits and The Mermaid and I have stripped down to swimming costumes. There are lugworm coils under my feet and when I touch the water the thrill is real after weeks of feet on dry land. A thousand knives jab at my skin as a heron eyes me beadily from a distance. The girls are squeaking and running away from the waves trickling over their toes, but I wade in and take a couple of strokes, rolling onto my back so that my shoulders are fully submerged. I'm gasping and smiling and high above me the waning Blood Moon is a gauzy surprise, still high in the sky after a long night of travel. The Littlest One asks me why the moon is still visible during the day and I don't have the answer. *Maybe you can be a scientist one day and explain these things to me* I suggest, but she shakes her head. *No Mummy, I'm going to be a disco farmer*.

When I look back at photos of that day now, there is a blurry one, an out of focus afterthought taken by The Whirlwind, where I am walking back out of the water with my arms outstretched to a shivering Caulbearer. Both of us are leaning in to each other, magnetically drawn because we belong in each other's arms, and it strikes me that at that moment I am fully grounded, the Earth to my daughter's moon.

We shuffle back to the cottage with towels draped around our soggy limbs, past a family dressed in warm coats and hats. *Your kids are braver than mine*, smiles the dad, and I don't know if that's true, but they are definitely brave. Deep down inside I hope that they feel able to be brave because they see me being brave. I feel frightened a lot of the time, but maybe that's what being brave is, doing things even though you are scared. Perhaps the rumbling terror that has pervaded these recent years can be reframed as an uncomfortable courage. I thank the man and walk on.

After a few days on our own my parents come to join us. The last time we were here the world was starting to shut down - we were only just beginning to understand that we could kill someone if we stood too close to them. This time we can breathe a little more easily, even if it is behind masks.

One day we decide to climb a hill. I have reassured The Mermaid that it is a short walk, that she can come back with me if it feels like too much, but I know this is a lot to ask. She brings a huge pink blanket with her and we start to climb. It's not a big hill, but it's windy and unknown, and lack of familiarity is always a challenge. Halfway up she tells me she has gone far enough. She curls up behind a cluster of rocks and hides underneath the blanket. I ask her if she is ok and she tells me she will lie down on the grass until we come back to collect her. She is very clear about what she can and cannot do, starting to put boundaries in place to protect herself and this feels like progress. She is determined beneath her blanket, safe to leave in the arms of the breeze for a few minutes.

The rest of us reach the top fairly quickly, scan the sea for Bass Rock and shout at my dad not to go too near the edge. The Whirlwind runs ahead, following a different path back down. Years of sharing a bedroom with her big sister have instilled a hypervigilance that I recognise in myself, an urgent need to check that The Mermaid is ok.

When we reach the rocks and the daughter under the blanket, another family is looking worriedly at us, concerned about the figure lying prostrate on the ground.

And yet The Mermaid is absolutely fine. She has navigated this walk in her own way, caring little, if anything, what anyone else thinks. And now The Whirlwind is chatting away to her grandad while The Caulbearer and The Littlest One argue about who will get to sit in the front on the way home. And I watch the four of them and realise we have not just climbed a hill, we have scaled a mountain.

By the end of the holiday I am still feeling lousy but these last weeks have felt like a lesson. Time spent in this cottage by the sea nourishes me. I have space to think, time to plan how to make our own little house nicer, press more of ourselves into it so it feels even more like home. Mum reminds me that I have always been like this, racing through life, crashing and burning. My illness is a heady mix of global pandemic, single motherhood, full-time caring and genetic predisposition. I might be changing, becoming more of the person I want to be, less scared, more thoughtful, but my brain still burns at a million miles an hour and my body has to deal with the fallout.

Back in Northumberland I stand on the landing surrounded by washing that needs putting away and many children who are not helping me. A cloud like a monster is hanging in the east. The moon is illuminated so I can see a perfect circle, but the Blood Moon is waning now, lying back, almost leaning on the rooftops. And then it is swallowed by the monster cloud and the sky goes dark.

11
Mourning Moon

Darkest Depths Moon,
Dark Moon, Snow Moon

One Sunday the younger girls are with their dad and I have to work. I am leading a singing workshop for women, helping them breathe their tensions out into the room and weave their voices into harmonies. Leaving all thoughts of children, ageing parents, work and a burning world at the door, I watch these women sink their bones into the floor, creases falling from faces. I tell them that this space is being held only for them, that everything else can wait, and then we sing together. I am good at these workshops, they combine my strengths: my creativity, musicality, teaching and extrovert nature. They bring out the best of me and I feel like I have been able to gift something special that these women can hold in their hearts when life gets messy.

I'm about to leave to drive to the hall where the workshop takes place, and I am moving my car onto the back lane so I can load my keyboard into the car. It is bulky and very heavy and I am still feeble from the virus, so I want to carry it as short a distance as possible. I drive up the street and turn onto the main road, planning to reverse down the lane. A tall man is walking along the pavement, so I indicate and wait for him to walk past. He strolls past my window and turns to look at me fiercely. I am not sure why he seems angry and check my mirror to see if I am blocking someone in. Everything seems fine but this man is still staring at me, intimidating me with the shadowy crevices on his face. I ignore him and reverse around the corner towards my back door, opening the boot and heading towards my house. I am not frightened, but I am unnerved, and I do not want this man to see which house I live in, so I turn back to my car and make a show of putting down seats and moving bags in the boot. I can see him walking across the top of the lane and looking at me once more, then he disappears from sight. Soon the keyboard is in the car and I shake the man from my head as I drive away, but wonder if I should have locked the front door because The Mermaid is inside and will she be safe.

Over the course of the afternoon I am distracted by singing and breathing, by melodies leaving lips and evaporating around me. I return home to a Mermaid engrossed in embroidery and burning a witch's brew of incense. A quick hoover around the house and then there are many little footsteps in the hall and my babies are all home. Poured through the door and into my arms.

I run a bath and fall into it, quickly soaping my hair before two daughters leap in with me. My legs are all twisted around the taps, head squashed uncomfortably against the tiles, but one day soon I will stretch my legs out in the hot water and wonder why the bath feels so big.

The sky outside is dark and I know it is smudged with cloud because there are no stars. The nascent Mourning Moon is nowhere to be seen, hidden somewhere out there in the night. With wet hair piled on my head and children skipping around in nighties, I ask The Mermaid to light the fire as I start on supper. She loves to do this, light matches and watch the paper disappear and the smoke rise. I feel as tired as it is possible to be as I chop garlic and pasta simmers, on some weird autopilot where senses are dulled but the mind is racing. We eat tomatoey pasta in bowls in front of the flames and watch a programme about toads. David Attenborough soothes us all with his hypnotic tones and the cat's fur is too hot to touch as she rolls on the hearth.

The Littlest One curls up on the sofa under a knitted blanket as The Mermaid picks up her embroidery once more. The Caulbearer sinks onto a cushion on the floor next to me and we fiddle with jigsaw pieces for a puzzle we have started. The Whirlwind chats intermittently and when we occasionally shush her she rolls her eyes and sighs. We are all together again and we are all safe, but my OCD is rearing its head. It flares up now and again, creeps up behind me when my guard is down. I am imagining the angry car man lurking outside our front gate and my brain won't allow me to realise I am catastrophising.

That's the thing about OCD, it is intense and extremely urgent, like a pressure cooker needing to let off steam. There is a jostle for control and rationale going on inside my head, but at times like this I struggle to find a way to manage it. The times when my brain is busy but my body is broken are the most dangerous, that's when the anxiety peaks. I send the girls up to get hot water bottles and start the usual night time routine. Stack the dishwasher and turn it on, pile up any pans and other bits that won't fit in the machine and leave them for the next load. Surfaces are wiped and I top up the cat's food and water bowls. Once the hot water bottles are filled I check the locks on the back door, scanning them several times with my eyes because one scan will not do. Sometimes I touch the locks because I need to make sure they are still cold hard metal, still up to the job of keeping us all safe. Then I go back into the kitchen and look at the knobs on the hob and the oven that must to be pointing to 12 o'clock. I like the lid on the piano to be down in case the cat jumps on it in the night and I think it is a murderer crashing about in my kitchen. Next I go back into the lounge, where sometimes I'll lift the blind my mum made for me, the one covered in berries and leaves, and touch the window latch, push it down so I know it is properly closed. I look at the glow of the embers in the fire and check there are not candles still burning. Finally, I go to my front door, where the real danger lies. I will almost always have locked this door some hours before, but I try the handle and jiggle it a bit. The door will not open. It is locked. Usually I will jiggle it once or twice more, then force myself to walk upstairs. But tonight once or twice more is not sufficient. I am regressing back to the days when everything is done in multiples of three and when I touch the handle I must be thinking of someone kind and safe. If I think of the angry car man when I touch the handle, he probably really is angry with me and he is probably outside, so I must start again with a different face behind my eyes and jiggle the door until I feel better.

This is OCD, this sense of another world racing through my head and removing me from reality. I have no idea why my brain has fixated on this man, and tonight I am unable to remember that my OCD appears when I am very tired. And I forget that the OCD means that my mind is too full of fear and that this is all happening because I need to be kind to myself and rest. All I know tonight is that if I don't jiggle my front door handle the angry car man will keep standing at my gate and looking up at my window and maybe he will even break into my house and steal my breath, break my children.

It is horrible, this fear, and it only subsides a little when I finally manage to leave my front door and climb into bed next to The Littlest One and read her a story about a duck and a mouse that live in a wolf's stomach. After that, The Caulbearer and I share a chapter in her Greek Myths book about Cronos swallowing his children. There are a lot of things being savaged tonight, not least my sanity. My gaze flickers backwards and forwards over the latches on the bathroom windows, until I see The

Whirlwind watching me suspiciously and realise that my madness is starting to show.

That night, after I have held all of my daughters close and wished them sweet dreams, I turn my light out and the darkness feels alive around me. I am like the mouse in the story, hiding under my duvet, waiting to be swallowed by the wolf.

The new moon started waxing five days ago but we have not yet seen it. Mourning Moon. The girls thought it was a Morning Moon, but it is nowhere to be seen when I step outside to take The Whirlwind down to her bus while everyone else sleeps. Instead the days are unfolding in a kaleidoscope of colours, burnished oranges and reds floating up from behind the rooftops. She tells me she watches the sky burn as she travels to school and I like to think about this after I have kissed her goodbye, her marble eyes reflected through the window.

When I go to wake up the little girls, tap my hand on the globe that will light up at my touch, the kaleidoscope is fading. *Good morning my babies* I say every time, and I lift their blind with lines of zebras and flamingoes and tell them that the sky is the colour of roses. If I am lucky, The Caulbearer will raise a sleepy head from the pillow and smile at the glow, though The Littlest One will bury her head deeper into her duvet and wait to be gently pulled from her dreams. If I am not so lucky, one of them will make a noise somewhere between a squeak and a groan, pin themselves to the sheets and refuse to get dressed. The Littlest One might sob loudly, cling to me as knotty hair sticks to wet cheeks, and I will have to cajole and cuddle them into their uniforms. You can never know what sort of morning it will be, but I can often rely on the backdrop to be a sky telling stories.

When we drive to the tiny school by the sea there is no Morning Moon, only horizons that seem wider each day, slashed with strips of white, like they have been clawed by a cat. The sun is low, barely above the tree line, and flocks of starlings erupt from the branches like ash. There are still trees like golden lollipops dominating the roads out of the town, and towards the coast gleaming hedges and skeletal branches create space so that the winter sun can creep through. At this time of year, as the days get shorter, I seek colour out in the skies. There are berries on the hawthorn, fields of deep green broken up by bright-eyed pheasants, but leaves are mulching into the ground, everything is hunkering down in anticipation of the frost that is surely only days or weeks away.

One Wednesday, I want to be at my desk, immersing myself in words and books and staring at candles, but I have promised my friend I will attend an autism support group. Sometimes, if The Mermaid is well enough to leave and the other girls are with their dad, I wake early on a Saturday and drive up to this friend's farm. In the summer, tourists park their cars along the verges of the road, walk a mile to the beach with surfboards on their heads and reusable bags spilling over with towels and spades, but the roads are empty whenever I arrive, except for the occasional hare loping across the field. My friend and I will run past the house I want to live in, a red brick beauty with a gable just before the dunes, and each time I will remind her that I am going to buy the house from her when I make my fortune. Then we run over the cattle grid, past the scrub of conifers on the left and the stables on the right, and we run up and down, between the sand dunes, until the path opens up onto Ross Sands, the most perfect beach I have ever seen.

Holy Island lies to the north, Budle Bay and Bamburgh to the south. We are sandwiched between castles and eyed by grey seals as we pound the sand and splash through the sparkle. When we reach the end of the beach we can come back via the oyster house, past the navigation points, and along the sandy path that skirts the fields. Or, more likely, we can turn around and run the way we came, stopping to strip off and run into the water, which will probably be calm and perfect and wrap itself around my body. I used to scream when I dipped in, while my friend glided out gracefully, a perfect reflection of her demeanour, but now I am used to the shock and just gasp quickly and roll over onto my back to gaze at the sky. Then we wade out of the sea, pull socks and trainers onto sandy feet and run back through the dunes to the farm.

This is the friend I have made a promise to, and it seems a small one in return for the magic she conjures on her beach. The support group is providing an opportunity for the local education authority to feed back on some report findings, and a senior figure from our children's mental health services will also be there. These two organisations have held my daughter's future in their hands for several years and I have a lot to say. We struggled to access the care we needed at our most vulnerable and I would like them to know that, though we are fortunate enough now to receive care from some excellent professionals. I have never found it in me to place a formal complaint about those who let us down, it feels like a misplaced use of my finite energy, but perhaps today I can share a sense of what families like mine need.

The Mermaid comes with me, wearing her grannie's heeled boots that make her feel bold, and slashes of black and crimson on her eyes and lips. She means business, and will later make me so proud when she raises her soft voice: her words are more powerful than any eloquent speech I might have prepared because this is her life. I can advocate and fight for her right to support and care, but I can never know what it is to experience life as she does. Only she can express that. She is more than a diagnosis, there is no one else like her, and she is always working hard to extract herself from the broad brushstroke society likes to paint her with. She doesn't want to be defined, just heard. The Mermaid often expresses herself in fabulous outfits she creates, through the cakes she designs and decorates, or as she dives under waves. Sometimes the words don't come. But today they do and I'm blown away by her power.

The village hall is full - mainly parents and carers, everyone fiercely advocating for someone they love who

deserves better. An older lady tells the story of her step-
son's diagnosis at the age of 35, asks why there is no
support in place for families like hers. Another woman
raises her hand and tells an almost identical story. There
are young mothers there who talk about teachers criticis-
ing their children's behaviour, children who are stressed
by noise or a change in routine and whose only crime is
to be misunderstood. There is a common theme of parents
not being listened to, of assumptions being made around
behaviour management and anxiety. I have been there
and I tell these two speakers just that. I wonder if they can
hear the impact of our experiences in my voice, which is
strong but charged with emotion. *I hear you* says the
man. *We have changed.* And I want to believe him.

The meeting goes on for over two hours, with The
Mermaid sitting next to me glamorous and poised, carefully embroidering a lily inside a small, circular wooden
frame. Needle in, needle out. When we stand to leave, I
hug my friend goodbye. *Well done*, she says. *Well done
both of you.* And the well done feels hugely inadequate
for what we have been through in recent years. The well
done should really be well done for still standing. Well
done for navigating a system that is broken. Well done for
holding each other tight. Well done doesn't cut it, but I
know what she means. Well done will do for now.

Northumberland is a splendid autumnal jewel as we
drive home. The sky is the blue of my daughters' eyes,
wisps of clouds like baby hair. The hills are burnished, a
deep purple where the heather is singing its last song

before the frosts arrive. The trees are majestic - we drive through tunnels of towering beeches and sycamores that remind me of the plane trees in Languedoc that I sailed under as a new wife. Those plane trees are diseased now and dying from canker stain, an incurable fungal infection that has resulted in thousand of trees being felled and burned. In 2005, when we sailed along the Canal du Midi, the infection was still dormant, no one knew about the tragedy that lay ahead. The fungus arrived with American soldiers during World War II, from the munition boxes they brought with them made from North American plane wood. We didn't know, as we chugged between locks, that we were helping the trees to die, chipping into the roots as we moored, tying rope around trunks and slicing into the bark, leaving them open to infection. So much we took for granted.

We went back there a few years later with the children, when The Littlest One was still a baby. They'd started cutting a small number of trees down by then. It was noticeable in patches, gaps where the sunlight had scorched the river bank and evaporated the water. I strapped my baby to my chest in a sling and cycled along the towpath with her small sweaty head nudging into my chest. The Caulbearer was in a little seat behind me, bobbing along on the back of the bike, and The Mermaid and The Whirlwind giggled in a trailer pulled by their dad, until one of them got dust in their eyes and we had to stop. It was possible to forget that the trees were dying if I kept cycling towards the shadows, parked up, balanced the bike against the fence and sat watching the light dancing on ripples left by boats. In those days I always carried raisins and biscuits, pieces of fruit and water bottles. There would be a baby on my breast, balancing against my knee, while I peeled a satsuma or unwrapped a cereal bar, child hands pawing my hair, soft cheeks nuzzling into my neck, and it would be hard to know where I ended and they began. Yes, it was easy to forget the trees were dying if I just kept cycling.

Daylight is trickling in through cracks in the cloud. The pavement is sparkling under street lamps, catching the shine of snail trails that run back and forth in front of me. I'm snowed under with university work and still not running because my energy levels are low. I start to wonder if running might improve things, shake off the constant headache I have had for the last few days, trigger some kind of miracle in my body that will shift the aftermath of this virus.

I can feel my impatience in the way I want to swallow the sky, gorge on its fiery reds and oranges until I am burning. I drop The Whirlwind off at her bus and I can see, just beyond the town where the fields become the sea, a sunrise so stunning that I consider driving until I reach it and diving into the sun-dipped waves. But instead I must turn back and wake the little two, brush their wispy hair into ponytails and pour milk onto cereal.

The mornings are getting darker still as we race towards the shortest day, weeks flying by so fast I can't catch them, life swirling past me and girls growing taller each time they fall into my lap. The Littlest One, in particular, has lost her chubby little girl look, all long arms and legs that drape themselves along sofas and against radiators, though her face is still cartoonish with full cheeks and eyes like pools you can drown in. I can see she is taller now than The Caulbearer, as they fold themselves into the back of the car and we set off on the school run.

Some days, often Fridays, they will want songs and we will sing our way to school. But both girls also like the quiet, some moments of calm before the day starts in earnest, and today is one of those days. Today the car is full of gasps and exclamations because the sun is rising in a blaze of glory. I keep stopping the car to take photos and stand in the chilly air. Everything has a burnished glow because the sun is dripping orange, gilding everything it touches. The girls are straining to look behind them. Autumn is breathing its last gasp and we are there to witness it.

Mummy come quickly! A stomping of feet on the landing above me and I know why they are calling. I run up the stairs where four excited daughters jiggle on tiptoes and point out of the window. The lights are off but the girls are bathed in a blueish glow, fairy hair shining, white nighties illuminated.

The Mourning Moon is beautifully waxing, more than half full and fierce enough to pierce the clouds hovering over the rooftops. We all stare up together and breathe in the night, bathe in the moonbeams and soak up the magic. Quite quickly, the moon will lift even higher above the town and we will all duck under the blind in the back bedroom. There is not room for us all, squeezing our knees onto the dressing-up chest under the window and catching our hair on the bells that dangle from the bunk beds, but we will all squash together and watch as the moon rises. It has hypnotised us all.

The next night I have finished tidying the kitchen after tea and upstairs everything is dark. Red and green flashes of light are popping out from under the door along with squeaks and shouts. The Caulbearer and The Littlest One are playing with a light sabre one of them was given at a party. It's only fun to play with when the lights are out and the game can end in tears. They burst onto the landing and spot the massive Mourning Moon, and all of a sudden we are spinning in moon glow and light sabre power and we stop, giddy, and look up at the sky. Beams of light, like a biblical arrival, are coming from the moon because we are staring so hard. There's a rainbow glow all around it, obliterating the clouds and dominating the sky.

I know that the girls have caught this moon obsession from me, from my constant gazing up and sighing, from the lunar calendar that hangs in my bedroom, from the hours I spend writing about moons. They start to tell me when they find a moon in a book, or a picture in a magazine. The Caulbearer's obsession with Greek Mythology continues and we discuss moon goddesses at length. The

Littlest One wants to know why the sun is brighter than the moon, why she can stare at the moon but not at the sun, and I cobble together a response supported by my very poor scientific understanding. The Whirlwind sends me photos of the sky on fire from her school bus, circling strange shaped clouds on the screen and asking me if I noticed them. And The Mermaid feels the moon in the tides, her fingernails turning purple because the water is colder now, but she needs the salt on her skin, the magnetic pull of the waves back to the shore. All of us are connected to each other by the moon, and now we have started to notice the sky there will never be a day when we don't look up.

As the days shorten, our life on the street becomes more insular. I go to the front door to call in the cat and stand on the step for a moment to see who is about. Builders mending a chimney a few doors down glance over at me. They glance a little harder at The Mermaid when she leaves the house in her clicky-clack boots and red lips. It is an uncomfortable feeling the first time a man turns his attention away from you and onto your daughter. I worry I am heading into the invisible years, feel conflicted that unwanted shouts from cars might stop and what does that say about me? The end of the 1990s was a strange time to come of age. I was endlessly confused by the concept of Girl Power, not realising until too late that it meant next to nothing because it only existed under the male gaze. I'm not sure any amount of feminism in the world will prepare me for the day I disappear from sight from half of the population; there is a definite conflict between wanting to be desired and objectification that is uncomfortable to unpick. For years my body was a vessel for my children, then a source of nutrition. In the last few years I have tried to prioritise its health and strength, but there are days when I wonder if the version of my body that is desired will ever resurface, whether I will even allow it to.

When the #MeToo movement was at its height, The Whirlwind asked me what it meant. When I told her, in eleven-year-old terms, she then asked if I had ever been assaulted by a man. I flinched at the question even coming out of her child mouth. And then I explained that there was a spectrum of assault, that every woman had experienced something on that spectrum and that micro-aggressions quickly become a white noise against which every woman and girl lives their life.

I didn't tell her about the time I was walking through Leicester Square, when a man reached up my skirt and grabbed at my knickers, his hand rough against my bare thighs. And I definitely didn't tell her about the evening I walked through an underpass, where a man opened his coat and glanced down, looked at me hungrily for a reaction before I ran away. I mentioned the time I was walking home from the pub with a friend and men shouted at us from a car, slowed down to match our speed as we hurried along, screeched off laughing when we ignored them and then drove up and down the road intimidating us until we hid behind a hedge with blood pumping in our ears. The

Whirlwind was with me when I was pushing The Caulbearer along in a buggy, eight months pregnant with The Littlest One, she was one of the two small daughters walking along beside me. She was with me when a horn sounded loudly just behind us, making us jump. She probably saw the men turning in their seats with twisted sneers on their faces, men who looked away when they saw my swollen belly. Soon enough she will know for herself what #MeToo means.

There are a couple of weeks this month when work becomes frenzied. I have lost over two weeks to isolation and illness and my days are still bookended with a sore throat that refuses to heal. At night I read with the girls, a story about owls with The Littlest One, more Greek myths with The Caulbearer, and the older two pop in and out of my room cuddling the cat or asking me to plait hair. Sometimes The Whirlwind likes me to read her poetry, or she will read a poem to me, tales of witches and dragon's breath. Words that float out soft and high in her child voice but carry all the power.

When everyone has been tucked up, I fall into a book of my own. My eyes are heavy and I'm fighting sleep but there will be more footsteps tiptoeing through, lights to switch off and fairy hair to stroke. I think that if I could sleep for a week, hibernate under the duvet and resurface after seven full days of rest I would be invincible. I am a terrible sleeper though, light as air, unable to fall into a deep slumber and stay there.

Despite my immune system having been battered, the stress, sadness and sleep deprivation are all woven into evenings like this and somehow alchemised into something good, with the blinds pulled down against a clear night sky and four daughters spinning like a carousel around the house. There is a symbiosis and calm in my tiny room, with the double bed squashed so firmly between the walls that the plaster is chipped and I will never be able to move house because the bed is stuck. The absolute horror and trauma of a family imploding is receding, waning like the moon, but occasionally felt in child tears on my neck, a flicker in The Mermaid's eyes and a book on the shelf that I still can't read because it was the last thing he gave me before we broke.

I am taking gentle walks to try and jump start my body back into life. One afternoon The Mermaid and I drive over to the school by the sea to collect the two little girls. We leave a little early, park at the hill that leads down to the beach and walk along a row of houses to a sunken patch of land behind the school. The quarry is backed onto by some new houses with weatherboard cladding clinging to the bricks, so you feel like you might be in New Zealand. Except this cladding is not wood but something else, composite maybe, and the landscape is unmistakably northern. It has rained heavily so the ground is claggy and branches glisten, dark against the berries that have almost all been eaten by the blackbirds and we can taste autumn on our tongues.

We pick our way down to the nature reserve, through mud that has been churned up by a truck. I'm tiptoeing on tussocks of grass because I put on inappropriate boots and the November air hurts my skin. The reserve lies between the beach and the new houses, a scrappy bit of land that has grown back into itself. Everything is bleached out by the winter light, lending a sepia glow to grass, reeds and low-lying hawthorn trees. Teasels diffuse the sun, their spikes entwining into a honeycomb effect that curves into moustaches. Two Exmoor ponies are eating grass where the land slopes up away from the lake, and I wonder why they are here. They remind me of ponies that used to walk across the roads when we crossed Dartmoor, driving from my childhood home in rural Devon to visit Granny and Grandad. I'm not sure what they are doing in Northumberland, or how they got here. Apparently after World War II only four Exmoor stallions remained in the world, only fifty ponies altogether. Even now there are less than 3000, and two of them graze on a patch of land behind my children's school, with a view across to the North Sea. There is a sign telling us not to disturb them, so we feel a bit like trespassers. The ponies lift their heads and assess our intrusion, but we are not enough to tear them away from the grass.

One Friday morning, as the Mourning Moon wanes, I wake before my alarm. The air in my bedroom is chilly. Night has not yet become a day that leaks through my blind. I roll over to check the messages on my phone.

There is often one from my sister that has arrived while I've been sleeping. I imagine her fresh from a shower and stepping out into her sun baked yard. It is so long since I have seen her, inhabited a space with her. To share the same air would be a gift. I don't allow myself to think too deeply about her physical absence in my life. I'd roll around inside the thought, get in too deep with it and I'm not sure I'd be able to extricate myself from the visceral pain of missing her. For the first few years after she left it was like someone had died: I was grieving all the times we would no longer spend together, the babies we would birth who wouldn't paddle in the same waves. And then I realised she wasn't coming back, and somehow it stopped hurting so much. It's the only time I've managed to build a wall around my heart, any other time it is there for the taking.

Just as I thought, like a delicious premonition, on my phone there is a message about Christmas parcels. I hear her voice like she is in the next room, press a heart emoji and send it to Australia.

Flick the lamp switch and bare feet on the floorboards. Twist hair on top of my head and put glasses on because it's too early for lenses. Pour myself into Grannie's dressing gown and hug myself as I wrap it around me. I've forgotten now those early mornings, when I would bury myself in his neck, soak into his warmth. Maybe that's another wall around the heart, something else best forgotten. Pad downstairs and hear a small cat shuffling behind the kitchen door. When I open it, she will curl herself around my ankles and trot down the hallway. I will open the front door, as I do every morning, and she will slip out into the postage stamp garden, hover next to the flower pot where she likes to torture mice, and then hop onto the wall.

The moon is just behind my rooftop so I can't see it. By the time I take the little girls to school in a couple of hours it will have swung around triumphantly into view and The Caulbearer will stand and stare at it for a moment before she gets into the car. Maybe looking for the hare. For now though, there are just perfect stars pricked into the night, and my feet are cold on the ground. I can breathe in the day that will soon creep in on a flame and watch until the cat slinks out of sight.

At the weekend Northumberland is hit by the worst storm for many years. Red warnings flash across the internet and our little pocket of the country is a headline for a few hours. We are usually lumped in somewhere between Tyne and Wear and the Scottish Borders, a forgotten world that has seen so many shifts between countries over the centuries, red skies mirroring blood-drenched soil. These age-old tussles over land feel exhausting, the obsession with possession and borders picking up momentum like a snowball and exposing everything that is ugly about humans. I wonder at what point did we begin to look at people as 'other', start to place ourselves into tiny boxes and arrange ourselves just so on the shelves?

I don't mean to be out in the storm. Mum texted me to check I'd seen the red weather warning and I have reassured her we will all stay safe. I text The Whirlwind asking her to take the bus straight home and email her drama teacher to say she can't attend the rehearsal after school. At 3pm I collect the little ones from the school by the sea and the children all run out into the playground laughing and sticking their tongues out to catch snow-flakes in the blizzard that is unfolding. At 4pm I wait for a call from The Whirlwind to say she is safely on the bus. Instead I receive an irate call from the bus driver asking where she is, he is waiting in busy traffic and he has other children to pick up. Then follows a frantic chain of phone calls between me, the school and the bus driver to try and establish where The Whirlwind has gone. Eventually the bus has to leave and I still have no idea where my daughter is.

A few weeks earlier she had come home from school telling me tales of men in a van shouting at girls in her year as they walked to school. 11-year old girls. The police were called and letters sent home to worried parents from the headteacher. I felt sick that the white noise of male aggression against women and girls, the white noise I feel as a prickle in the back of my shoulders or a lurch in my chest, had now spread to another gener-ation, and my daughters would have to develop tactics of their own to cope with it. Inevitably the advice coming from the school was not to walk alone between school sites, to report anything suspicious. I told The Whirlwind to step back from any cars that pulled up close to her, walk away if a car slowed and someone spoke to her.

And then I hated myself for planting a fear that might not have existed, and I told her it was not ok that women and girls are forced to change their actions because of the bad behaviour of some men and boys. I told her not to be scared, just safe, but I knew that by having this conversation I had opened a miserable can of worms.

It is against this backdrop that I momentarily lose my daughter, then discover fairly quickly that she has in fact gone to the rehearsal and must not have received my message. The next problem is that the rehearsal is taking place in the city, and the route to collect her is directly in the path of the storm.

These are the situations when being a single parent is challenging. I look around the bedroom, where there are children in various states of undress, wrapped in towels with hair dripping onto the carpet. In the doorway stands The Mermaid, immediately picking up on my own anxiety, flickering her eyes from left to right and saying *what shall we do Mummy*? I have very little choice but to throw everyone into onesies, grab my phone and head out into the storm, potentially putting us all in danger of being squashed by a tree or skidding into a snow drift. The Caulbearer doesn't like being in the car when it is dark so I strap her into the front seat, show her where the sweets are hidden and turned Disney Hits on loudly to drown out the wind that is whistling between the roof bars. The Mermaid and The Littlest One cower in the back seat, huddle under a blanket and it feels like we are on a rescue mission. The snow has stopped, there are no trees flying across the road and I manage to make it fun, pointing out strands of fairy lights being whipped by the wind. In the city the girls stare at more festive decorations, red lights from traffic jams illuminating the puddles. We pull into the school car park and wait for The Whirlwind. One of the girls has found an awful playlist which alternates between S Club 7 and McFly, but at least it disguises the wailing of the storm, which is getting louder.

At last a white-blonde pony tail bounces towards us and The Whirlwind collapses into the back seat, blithely unaware of any drama and demanding to know what's for tea. It is rush hour now and the SatNav is indicating a different route back to the A1. We reverse out of the carpark and I follow the instructions down streets of red brick houses with shiny black gables and matching bay windows. The girls are all chattering and I am keeping my eye on the map on the screen. The long residential street that leads to the main road is lined with parked cars so that there is not much space. A grey 4x4 is driving towards me, not intending to stop, and I look ahead for a space to pull into to create room for it to pass. I turn into a gap between the parked cars and look across at the 4x4 to make sure it has room. The 4x4 is only inches from me, and I look up into the driver's window where a furious man has jammed his middle finger against the window and is staring at me with a look of angry disdain.

My immediate response is to make light of the situation, so I smile at him and give him a thumbs up. I don't know that ignoring is the best form of defence, I always want a happy ending. To be honest I am shocked that he is angry at all - I have given way to him, I am trying to help him get past. The man continues to gesticulate at me and mouth obscenities, and now the girls have noticed and I just start saying *you are being so rude* and pointing at my four children sitting all around me. I try to pull in further. The man's face is white and pinched, his mouth tight. His anger is all contained inside the 4x4 but he is pushing his finger hard against the window as if he wants to reach right through the glass and show me just how cross he really is. I am still asking him to stop, showing him I am trying to move over and could he please not be abusive in front of my daughters, but as I edge forwards and enable him to finally pass he flings one last gesture at me, his words swallowed by the storm, and speeds away down the street.

The whole incident can't have lasted for more than thirty seconds, but I am shaking for a long time afterwards. Feeling wobbly as I turn onto the main road, telling the girls I should have got his number plate because that was unnecessary and surely illegal, and The Mermaid straight away parrots the licence number to me because her memory is amazing. A personalised number plate. A rich man in a big car swearing at a woman and four girls for driving down a street. Later that night I go onto the maps app on my phone to see if I had inadvertently gone the wrong way down a one-way street, as if that might have justified being abused in my own car. I hadn't as it turned out. I was just getting in his way.

I can't think about him now though because the storm has really picked up. Heading north on the A1 I can't see the lines on the roads because snow is sweeping across the windscreen and I'm holding on tight to the steering wheel against massive gusts of wind. The girls in the back are saying *well done Mummy, you can do this, we are nearly home*! And I am saying *don't worry girls, we can do this, nearly home*! We are great cheerleaders for each other. The Caulbearer in the front seat has wide eyes reflecting the tail lights ahead and her face is as pale as the snow hammering the car. A couple of miles to the east the North Sea is smashing into the beaches, each wave dragging the sand back, claw-like, and hurling it back at the coastline, fierce and unrelenting. Later that night thousands of trees will be slammed to the ground, taking power lines down and cutting us off from the world. But first I will slowly indicate, drive down to the roundabout and turn left onto the road that takes us home. I will open the car door, feel myself being sucked from the car, unlock the front door and shout for my daughters to run inside. I will light the fire, cook pizzas in an oven, pour orange squash for them and a glass of red wine for me. I will force the clattering letterbox down with useless strips of sellotape and listen as The Whirlwind tells me there are things falling down the chimney. *It's just the storm*, I tell her, *we are all safe. Mama's here.*

12
Cold Moon

Oak Moon, Moon Before Yule,
Long Night Moon

The rooftops are kissed with a white sheen, a layer of ice that will slowly shrink as the sun moves higher and people inside the houses turn up their thermostats. Some days the sky is on fire and The Littlest One will swivel around in the car to tell me *it is chasing us Mummy*! *The fire is chasing us!* On those days I drive home from school via the coast, carefully step out of the car and tread onto shiny puddles with leaves trapped beneath frozen surfaces. The sky falls into a sea with waves that ripple pink onto the sand, and the air clings to my cheeks until they too are rosy, and my fingers are numb against the screen of my phone. The pictures I take can never reflect the stun I feel standing above the beach staring across to the horizon. But still I take photos, as if I can store some of the sea's power in my phone and save it for later. Draw on it when I really need some magic.

* * *

My post-viral malaise has developed into yet another illness, a livid rash under my arm that weeps and stings. Shingles. I text a friend to tell her I can't meet up with her and she nails it: '...*an indication you are doing too much. But who else will do it?*'

And there it is. Who else will do it? I am blessed with beautiful, supportive friends and family. My parents and my brother will care for The Mermaid so I can escape for a night or two. Neighbours and local friends showed up daily on the doorstep when she was in hospital and during our various isolations. Faraway friends and siblings send messages and little parcels, check in with me if I go silent. The girls' schools hold my daughters close, offer them hope and distraction from a home that has sometimes been fraught with illness, sadness and fear. We are looked after by a community that wraps its arms around us, and yet I still need to learn to look after myself because underneath everything lies an ever-present fear that one day I will be too ill to care for my children.

So much of my life comes down to fear. I have spent too long being scared. Scared of ending my marriage. Scared of losing my children. Scared of what people think. Scared of making mistakes. Scared of not living life to the full. Scared of not giving my daughters the childhoods they deserve. Scared of men shouting at me from cars. Scared of being with men. Scared I will never know how to be with a man again. Always scared.

But as the rash under my arm heals and my body is returned to me, the grey haze that has been draped miserably over the last few weeks begins to lift. Sometimes I hover above this woman, wonder if she is good enough, if this is what a good parent looks like, what a good person looks like. This woman who has chosen to no longer stand in the background, who persists in challenging individuals, argues with authorities that have tried to force her voice back into her throat. At times it has felt like her breath has been stolen, but she is one of the lucky ones. Her breath was there all along, gently blowing away wisps of fairy hair as she held small daughters close. Murmuring in the ear of a child immersed in another world, softly bringing her back. And sometimes her breath is a roar, a guttural moan that can't be ignored, a cry commanding attention.

She is one of the lucky ones.

Under the Mourning Moon I had intended to run in an endurance event through the Cheviot Hills - another grand gesture, wild weather and a body pushed to the limit. I've never done that distance before off-road, and I wanted to know what it would feel like to be both vulnerable and strong out on those hills, as perhaps I am every day of my life amongst the preparation of pasta and the washing of clothes. But my body has other ideas so, searching for a way to thank Northumberland for the skies I have lost myself in and the waves I have found myself in, I somehow create a child-free window and plan a sunrise walk.

I set an alarm and wake while the sky is still dark. It is the day before the winter equinox so light is at an absolute premium. I make myself a cheese sandwich and a thermos of coffee. Pack a bottle of water and an apple, my notebook and pen. It is not particularly cold for the time of years, but I have my long coat, scarf and gloves because the wind chill might trick me.

I leave The Mermaid for a few hours because she is going to work at a café in town. A lovely woman has learned about her passion for baking and asked if she can help her to develop these skills. And so every week now The Mermaid will go to this little café that serves hot chocolate in pink cauldrons, and she will begin to build a life that is just for her. The effort it takes to paint on her smile and walk alone into town is huge, but once she arrives she can whisk the world away and mould magic from sugar. The stable moments where I can worry less are becoming more frequent. I can never rely on them, need always to be prepared to change or cancel plans, but today The Mermaid sleeps sweetly and when I kiss her goodbye she is happy to be left and take herself off to the café. Contrast this with last year when I could barely leave her in a room on her own and it's the only Christmas present I need.

The sky clings to the rooftops as I get into the car. Any hopes I had for a world exploding into life are dashed - today the day will crawl in like a reluctant child. As I drive up the A1, the only colours glowing amongst the drabness are the line of taillights I am following north and the level crossings of the railway line up to Scotland. In the spring this stretch of road is perfect for spotting hares and deer in fields, or buzzards hanging on thermals. Today the landscape is muted, the lightening of the skies barely noticeable. The opposite of a grand gesture.

After about twenty minutes on the road I glance across to the east, where the North Sea lies like a ribbon. The skyline is broken up by Bamburgh Castle, and I imagine the rock pool just beyond it where I have swum so many times this year. North of Bamburgh the beaches are white and wide, and now a mass of land is emerging through a sky the colour of dirty dishwater. Another castle hangs on the end of this mass, and just a little south The Farne Islands begin to emerge. This is Lindisfarne, or Holy Island as it is perhaps better known, where St. Cuthbert used to treads the sands. Today I am going to drive across the causeway while the tides are low and walk around the island, try to feel what it is to be alone on an island famously linked to solitude and retreat. I will be circling the island while the tides are low so that I can nip back across the causeway before it closes. For a real sense of isolation I should wait for the tides to rise so that the island is separate from the mainland once more. But true isolation is not possible in the absence of long chunks of childcare, so I must make do with a sunrise escapade and be back in time to collect The Mermaid before lunch.

The causeway is flanked by mud flats, its tarmac road barely visible under sand that has blown across it during the recent storms. Wooden poles mark the walking route taken by pilgrims just a little to the south of where I am driving. A redshank pecks in the mud and further out I spot the unmistakeable curve of the curlew's beak. The sky is lightening imperceptibly, and there will be no grand gestures for me this morning. The Cold Moon is submerged in cloud so that I feel genuinely alone, no satellite to guide me.

I park the car and head back towards the causeway where a footpath should take me across the dunes towards the North Beach. A woman and an older couple are throwing a ball for a dog but otherwise there is no one about. It's light now, but the type of light where windows glow orange and if you were inside it would still look dark outside.

As I walk along the road I hope I will hear the ghostly moan of seals from the sandbanks, like wind whistling through roof bars. It's quiet though, the air weirdly still and only broken up by curlews bubbling in distant fields, geese honking and a lively cockerel. When I reach the footpath sign it is barely visible amongst many cows, who have congregated by the fence. They stare at me mournfully with their creamy faces and dappled bodies and I know I will not be taking that route today. I continue walking back towards the causeway and hope for another path.

A greylag goose lies dead on the flattened grass, strangely beautiful with its neck bent back and wrapped around its body, like a ballerina with its pink beak stretching out. Its eye is closed, not yet savaged by crows, and I imagine its body might still be warm if I stroked it. I stand and look at the goose for a long while, wonder if I could be inhaling the last breath from its body, catching it as it floats up from the ground before it disappears into the air.

Just beyond the goose I spot a hole in the wire fence with a makeshift path winding through the marram grass. If I throw my rucksack through and crouch down low I can crawl under the wire. I do this and gaze north where I know the sea is waiting beyond the dunes. The marram is soaked in mud and rainwater, flattened in places, and here and there hawthorn trees rise from the ground like twisted spines, stripped of berries so no colour, just gleaming silhouettes against the smudged sky.

As I walk away from the road, night has somehow crept into day without any kind of fanfare. During the winter months in Northumberland most of the colour can be found in the sky, in explosive sunrises that force me to my doorstep or a world on fire as we arrive home from school. Today the morning has arrived cautiously, mirroring my steps as I tiptoe over marshy ground in ancient walking boots. Three roe deer are chewing grass less than a hundred metres away and I whisper to them softly, carefully edging past and trying not to frighten them. Their white bottoms are a welcome flash of brightness in the gloom, cartoon ears silhouetted against the dunes.

The North Sea is concealed from here, hidden by dunes that rise and fall. The only indication that I will soon stumble upon a beach is a sky stretching up to Cuthbert's heavens and a distant rumble that can only be waves swallowing sand. I round a dune and come eye to beady eye with a heron that immediately takes flight, a dinosaur bird creaking its way into the air. Ahead of me I see two people walking with their dog and feel relieved when they climb over a stile taking them back towards the village. During the summer months tourists pour onto the island as the tide ebbs to reveal the causeway. I don't consider myself a tourist, I've lived nearby for almost ten years. For a long time I was a city-dweller, ending up alone in Northumberland with my children by accident or fate. I have worked hard to love my home, pounded its earth, tumbled in its waves, written endless love letters to its wide skies, but my heart can still leap or lurch depending on my mood.

The sky is brushed with apricot as a thin strip of steely sea emerges beyond the marram, and the world is a little lighter as I stare towards Scotland. It's fresher too up here, a little more alive, and it's a relief to leave the strange stillness of the dune lands. Today the beach has formed a crescent, its contours pummelled by Storm Arwen a few weeks earlier. A large pool of water has formed on the sand as oystercatchers call and a black-backed gull looms above me. It's peaceful enough, a living breathing Turner painting, but the relentless dragging of the tide is ominous, a reminder of the many ships that have been tossed onto this beach and further out onto the rocks of the Farne Islands. Along this stretch of the island, the low-lying cliffs have been savaged by the weather, ripped away until they are just scars.

The sky is becoming luminous with the promise of something. Clouds are drenched with sun but still too thick to offer more than a gleam as I walk east towards Emmanuel Head, a white brick pyramid daymark built at the beginning of the 19th century to guide ships to safety. Despite its efforts, around seven hundred lives have been lost in this fierce pocket of sea, lending the island's reputation for peace and calm a sinister edge.

As I pick my way through a flock of sheep that has drifted onto the footpath I look down to the shoreline. The sun is starting to peer through the cloud and a heron's shadow is black on the glossy water. I walk past a hawthorn tree bent almost horizontal by the wind, hunched over like a prickly old man. It's bleak here, brutally exposed to the elements. The sand below shudders at memories of warrior cries, sighs at the stolen breath of sailors. I pull my scarf a little tighter around my neck, wondering if it is possible that the irony of Holy Island is that it is impossible to be alone. This feels like a place where ghosts can congregate freely. Rather than an hermitic retreat, if you listen carefully Holy Island is busy with voices floating through the air, weaving themselves into future generations.

Walking down from the castle, I'm following the perimeter of the harbour towards the village. Wooden staithes stand alert amongst the stones and the seaweed, and my eye follows the stretch of water over to the twin beacons at Guile Point. A group of tourists are taking photographs, and as they laugh they miss a curlew flying across from the water and landing in a nearby field. *Hello curlew*, I whisper, and once more I am not alone. I'm cold though, fingers bitten by a brisk December breeze and a streaming nose. Someone has lit a bonfire. I breathe in the smoke and stare at coloured boats called *Sea Witch* and *Cowbar Lass*.

This scrap of beach strewn with seaweed is littered with fishing paraphernalia - lobster pots stacked like barrels, ropes and hoses coiled on gravel, and plastic crates to be filled with fish and ice then sold on. Herring boats are turned upside down for storage, while nets and ropes hang from a nearby tree. Above the adorned tree lies The Heugh, a long flat-topped rock that forms a natural barrier between the old church and monastic buildings and the sea.

I have climbed down to the rocky beach below the Heugh with my children many times, where we spot glossy seal heads poking out of the water, and pocket pieces of sea glass like milky emeralds or pearly mussel shells. Once we walked around to Hobthrush Island, a tiny piece of land connected at low tide, five girls in wellies exploring the edge of the world. I don't walk across to it today, but I stare at it for some time, remembering that day when we sat in a grassy hollow sketching flowers and the realities of life seemed a million miles away.

I must return to the rest of the world now before waves fold over the causeway and leave me stranded. On my way back to the car though I wander through the graveyard of St. Mary's Church, humble in the shadow of the ruined priory, with its rosy Borders stone. The graves are blown almost bare by the weather, lettering faint and crusted with lichen. Some of the stones are cold and bumpy to touch with no indication of who might be buried beneath. But I manage to pick out the names of Thomas Kyle, coxswain of Holy Island, and Marian Bell, the postmistress, and I can't help feeling once more that this is an island of people. The power of the place lies in its ability to make us feel that we are never alone, to diminish our fears and worries and remind us that our lives are just tiny moments in time. My whispers will be added to the winds whipping this little corner of Northumberland, joining a chorus of voices from long ago.

One night I have a dream. I am in a speedboat on the Thames with my ex-husband's family. The Littlest One is sitting on my knee but she is a baby. The boat is low down in the river so that we are level with the water, which is turquoise and translucent, strangely cloudy as particles dance in the sun. I am holding on tightly to The Littlest One but she slips from my grasp and I watch her float away, fall beneath the surface and out of my reach. As so often happens in dreams, I cannot move, my voice is swallowed. But before the horror can really take hold, a couple swimming in the river catch my daughter and pass her back to me, and the dream moves on.

We arrive at the last week of term before the schools break up for Christmas. The headlines are a blur of political corruption and a pandemic spinning out of control. One morning I find myself swearing at the radio after dropping the little girls off, wondering why charlatan is such a pretty word for such ugly behaviour. I take the scenic route home in order to watch the sun rising above a fractious sea, its glow dripping into the water like a majestic puddle.

We are nearing the shortest day, barely eight hours of daylight in this northern corner of Britain. When I wake each morning and creep downstairs to let the cat out, the sky is either a swirl of cloud, smudged like charcoal into paper by The Caulbearer's careful fingers, or a witch's cloak, inky and pricked with stars. The moon is nowhere, sunken below the horizon, making its journey to visit my sister, who is now roasting in temperatures of over forty degrees. Yin and yang, hot and cold, light and dark. None exists without the other, and perhaps we are both drawn to extremes, tiny dots orbiting in opposite hemispheres.

The school run now begins in darkness, child faces wiped clean of milk and honey are caught in the glow of the dashboard. We look up at street lamps that fizz and blur in our vision, enjoy the Christmas lights shining out from houses. A strip of purple and fuchsia clings to the horizon, slowly rising until the sky in the west is flecked in baby pinks and blues. Blackbirds are captured in the headlights, skittering between the hedgerows, and when we stop at the level crossing, tired heads loll against windows. As I drive away from the school, daughters safely in their classrooms, the sea is a steely blue swathe, stubborn and constant. I reluctantly turn away and head home.

The Mermaid continues to walk on her own to the cafe, lips painted red, long skirt kissing her ankles, just comfortable enough to inhabit both her body and her mind. She is pale but happy when I collect her at the end of her short shift, and I know that the effort this outing takes will show itself in the evening.

One night I have just climbed into bed. The Littlest One has been asleep for a couple of hours, her long body growing as eyelashes rest on her child cheeks. The Caulbearer and The Whirlwind are tucked up with books and I'm about to delve into one of my own.

The Mermaid appears at the door, eyes darting from side to side and a waterfall of unspoken words ready to tumble from her lips. Mothering four daughters requires me to listen endlessly, to hear difficult words and respond as wisely and carefully as I am able, though every day is new for me too. The end of a sixteen-hour day, when I am exhausted and relying on a book to take me into another world, is not a good time for deep discussions. But inevitably this is often when The Mermaid needs me most, and I must try to rise to the occasion.

Tonight, she tells me that ever since she can remember it has felt as if everyone else in the world is blue, and she is yellow. Her voice is faltering and cracking and her face is streaked with tears. I call to The Whirlwind to bring through a blanket, and she rushes in, knowing the drill, and hands over an old woollen throw. I smile at her as she trots back to bed, fleetingly wondering how she will talk about her childhood when she has grown, what the impact will be upon her of having a mother whose attention must so often be elsewhere. And then I wrap my oldest daughter up and she rocks gently backwards and forwards on her knees, her eyes fixated on the coloured fairy lights that hang beside my bed. I tell her that it is fine for her to be yellow and the rest of the world blue, that she must learn to love being yellow and celebrate her otherness. I tell her that most people feel other, that everyone wears a mask sometimes, and then I worry that I am belittling the challenges she experiences in her life. But I glance up at her face and it is as if she is still the little girl who collected helicopter seeds in the playground. Her skin is still smooth, her forehead gently sloping down to meet her beautiful hazel eyes, and I wonder who was that little girl, did I ever really know her? I start to scan back over her life to search for clues that I missed the first time around. Her otherness has always seemed perfect to me, but I am not her and I do not experience life the way she does, like an explosion of fireworks in her head. The other day she told me that when she comes to my choral concerts she sometimes hears the music as white noise, with no disparity between the different voices. It's not unpleasant, she reassures me, but she doesn't think it's what everyone else hears.

Her breathing has slowed down now, the blues and reds of the lights faintly glowing on her skin. She feels able to return to the bedroom she shares with The Whirlwind, just next door and I hope I have been enough.

For many children, the Christmas celebrations enjoyed at school are exciting, an opportunity to wear brightly coloured jumpers instead of uniforms and watch Elf whilst making endless paper chains. The Littlest One falls into this camp, singing about stars above stables as we drive past skeleton trees leaking red through their branches. The Nativity soundtrack is played on a loop as she bounces around on her booster seat.

The Caulbearer is another story, and as the term draws to a frenetic close she runs into my arms at the school gates with a pale face. In the car on the way home, The Littlest One chats and chats about what she had for lunch, how many points she got on her maths test, how she was chosen to make popcorn and it exploded all over the place, how her teacher wasn't in today so another teacher was in charge. It's an effort for anyone else in our car to get a word in edgeways, and as I navigate the familiar roads I look in the mirror and watch The Caulbearer leaning her chin on her hand and gazing out of the window to watch the sky turn golden.

In the evenings she is straight into her purple koala pyjamas, barely talking, but underneath I imagine her brain is ticking like an engine, pistons banging and crowded conveyor belts refusing to stop.

One night I am cooking tea - spaghetti bolognese maybe or macaroni cheese, a staple meal that I can make with my eyes closed, or at least whilst doing about seven other things at the same time. The Caulbearer is hovering next to the kettle, bare feet shuffling on the laminate floor, brow furrowed, blue eyes dipping down under long lashes. I ask her if she wants to help me. *I don't know*. Would she like me to find her something to do? *Don't know*. Her little face is contorted, struggling with something she would like to articulate but the words aren't coming. I am reminded of the time The Mermaid's teacher told me she never spoke in class, and me later discovering that this was because she could not listen and speak at the same time, the processing was just too much. But I tuck this memory away, another memory of being told I am making my child anxious pushing its way to the front. Somewhere along the way, intuition and empathy became neurosis and paranoia in the eyes of the people I needed to listen.

The Caulbearer should be at a dance class this evening, but the plans all got mixed up and this confusion was too much for her after a day of being an angel and wearing a tinsel headdress that itched and wondering what had happened to her normal timetable and why she was in a different room, not her classroom. The staff at school rarely see much of the fallout, just the odd morning when I have to coax her out of the car and carry her to the door because everything is overwhelming. She's fine after you've gone, they tell me in brief emails, meaning to reassure me. But I am just reminded of the ghost in the subtext I used to hear when The Mermaid's teacher told me the same: she's fine after you've gone (because you are the problem). Like I say, empathy becomes paranoia.

I hold my arms out to this little daughter, lift her up to my chest. Her body is tense but not resistant and she wraps herself around my neck, legs clinging to my waist. *Is there something inside you needing to come out?* She nods. Holding on to my tiny girl, who is frail and warm in my arms, I look for a song on my phone, one we can spin to, one that we love. I find the Pas de Deux from Tchaikovsky's Nutcracker (I can be festive as well as therapeutic) and the harp's arpeggios fill the kitchen. As the cellos soar I cuddle The Caulbearer and spin round and round, socks slipping on the floor. Her head is buried deep into my neck, her white blonde hair tangled up in my long brown knots and we are twirling fast as pasta bubbles on the hob. Slowly I can feel her unfurl and her body relaxing into mine.

I inhabit a world of strong feelings and emotions expressed through words. I have an intense desire to understand, unpick, explain, explore everything verbally, through sentences that roll through my head, and this trait is not one that is always shared by The Caulbearer and The Mermaid. Sometimes words aren't helpful.

The strings are rising now and any moment a cymbal will crash. Right on cue, The Littlest One, drawn by the noise of the orchestra, bursts through the door and demands to join in. The Caulbearer is smiling now, her eyes shining once more. We hold hands in a circle and spin, pirouetting as we fall away into corners of the kitchen, laughing and breathing into the room. Something about the movement has dislodged the anxiety swirling around my daughter's head, something more primal that comes from her very core, and once more her words can spill out when she needs them. She is pink-cheeked now, glowing under the fairy lights draped around the kitchen table, running to find her bouncy hopper and squealing with her sister.

I turn back to the pasta and watch the water swirl.

As much as I'm a sucker for the grand gestures, sometimes the day will roll in gently and that can be just the balm I need. It's the last day of term and I wake before the alarm. Many, many mornings of rising early to work or drive a small daughter to her bus have become part of my fabric, and now these moments before the girls wake and the day cranks up are precious and only for me.

I pad downstairs to let the cat out, wait to feel her long tail winding itself around my legs and flick on the kettle in the kitchen, last night's plates carefully stacked and waiting to be loaded into the dishwasher. Back along the hallway the floorboards are cool under my feet, and when I unlock the front door the mild air of recent days has gone, pushed out by a weather front that has spread frost on the grass and ice on windscreens. The sky is endless black, stars pulsing and blurring in my gaze, and the cat has slipped through the cast iron gate and trotted down the road. Across the street, fairy lights twinkle in the neighbour's windows, and I know that as I close the door behind me the one opposite will open to reveal a man and his tiny toy poodle on a lead. The to and fro of life, bare feet on icy doorsteps, cats slinking around ankles, steam rising from endless cups of tea. Day after day punctuated by these small routines, yet somehow everything is changing. I am changing.

I wake The Caulbearer and The Littlest One and they climb out of bed, one by one folding themselves into my lap like cats, warm and sleepy. I hang their uniforms on the heater and slip toasty clothes over their pale little bodies, tempting them with *what will be in your advent calendar this morning* and *would you like some honey?* I carefully smooth knotty hair into bobbles, ignoring the opportunities to brush out the tangles because that will be a step too far on a dark December morning. From the front these two girls look as neat as pins, almost the same size so that they are often mistaken for twins. On occasion, when walking in a trio with The Whirlwind, they are mistaken for triplets to their absolute horror, The Mermaid standing apart from them with darker hair and her mother's eyes.

We head out to the car, the girls with tummies full of milk and bagels, breath evaporating into the winter air and steaming up the windows. The day is the colour of peach bonbons with streaks of baby pink ripping up the sky, the horizon silhouetted like a shadow theatre, dark trees glossy and wrapped in overcoats of ivy. When we arrive at the little school by the sea I hold the hands of my two littlest daughters, *come on my Christmas hens* I say, and they erupt into giggles. *Why are we hens Mama?* I have no idea why they are hens, but as I kiss their foreheads and they trip through the door my chest is clenching because I couldn't love them any more than I do at that moment, watching their blonde heads disappearing behind the glass.

After days of skies that are ripped open like my heart broken and bleeding onto the land, a smoky veil drapes itself over the rooftops and the world feels a little smaller. The full Cold Moon is due to rise at the weekend but our tiny town is submerged in gloom, the sun sunken in thick cloud, air stagnant and stubborn. There are no grand gestures, no fizzing stars blinking at me as I open the front door each morning, and I resort to burning candles, lighting the fire and staring into the flames.

There are no children in pyjamas hopping on the landing and yelling at me to look at the sky because the youngest three have gone to stay with their dad for five days. The house is filled with echoes, dust revealing itself as I climb the stairs, catching the slight breeze from my movement and reminding me of tumbleweed. Earlier today I drove the girls, shiny clean and dressed in Christmas jumpers, down to the city where some of his family were waiting. I bumped into them outside the flat and hoped that the stars on my cardigan made up for the sadness in my soul. Held on tightly to The Littlest One as she clung to my neck, kissed her and hoped a little bit of me would stay with her until I could hold her again. Picked up The Caulbearer, light as a fairy, and said *I love you* into her ear, imagined the words travelling deep inside her and keeping her warm during the nights I couldn't tuck her in. Rocked her as I remembered that

words don't always work for that daughter. Breathed in
The Whirlwind's hair as she wrapped her arms around
my waist and dismissed the thought that she is too big
now to carry in my arms, waved it all away as I walked
out of the flat and the door closed behind me.

The Mermaid is wrestling with the broken shards of her
fragmented family, trying desperately to make sense of
her world. She comes to me frequently asking for a cuddle
and I can see her brain working too hard to manage the
change. Despite this, she is able to take herself off to do a
shift at the cafe, painstakingly painting glitter onto
biscuits, finding solace in the intricacy of her work, creating something a bit more perfect.

The first Christmas we visited the beach, it was covered
in starfish. The timing was perfect, stars scattered across
the sand. But it meant that every year after that, when the
only treasures to be found were razor shells and sea glass,
the children wondered where the starfish had gone. It was
an absence - a small one, but it highlighted the huge one
looming over us all.

Once there were six of us, stuck together with a glue
that was four windswept daughters. If I close my eyes
now I see skinny legs in tiny wellies, child cheeks raw
from the cold. A man in a grey coat, not quite tucked in,
fraying at the edges. The sky was winter pale. Maybe the
sun shone, but in my memory it was a day stripped of
colour, the backdrop to a melodrama. A soundtrack of

soaring strings would have worked well, but instead, there were gulls and oystercatchers, and the thrill of delighted children as more and more starfish appeared.

Later, the beach didn't looked the same. Not in the way that it never looks the same because each tide carves a different pattern, slicing into the estuary at new angles, forming slopes and pools that move with every moon. Not like that. It never looked the same because we were not the same. We were only five now. The wellies were a little bigger, the child cheeks perhaps just as pink, but now the person fraying at the edges was me.

A couple of years ago we went to a different beach. There was a gloss on the sand, and the sun threw patterns on the waves. I was thinner but my heart was fuller, freer somehow. There's a photo somewhere of the five of us, and I believe the smiles on our faces. They were real.

Three missed calls from the girls' dad and my heart is trying not to race as I ring him back. The Caulbearer has fainted, has a fever and a couple of spots on her face. Immediately I think it must be chicken pox she has caught from my hefty bout of shingles and ask if he wants me to drive down and collect her. But he is fine, she is fine, and there is a speck of solace in occasionally being able to work together and do the best for our children.

The Mermaid has been flickering between the world in her head and reality, and I have needed to work harder to pull her into the day. Her turmoil is experienced viscerally, throughout all parts of her body as she shakes and clings to me. *There is a thought in my head that won't come out* she whispers, and I want to crawl inside her brain and stroke it, massage it until the horror evaporates. But the thought is trapped and all I can do is hold her, spin a spell with my words, hope they will soothe her. It occurs to me that last Christmas The Mermaid was only just out of hospital, could not walk. I didn't know it then but her head was starting to spiral out of control and I was losing her. Maybe the fairy lights and glitter at this time of year remind her of the days when she started to get lost in the dark.

One more sleep and the girls are home. The Caulbearer is a whisper of a girl, pale and poorly as she stumbles from the car into the house and when I lift her up there are tears down her cheeks as she clings to me with her legs. The Whirlwind and The Littlest One are full of the presents they have been given and *I can't wait until Christmas Eve Mama*. The girls' dad walks back to his car and I try not to wonder if he will be spending Christmas alone. The Mermaid stands quietly by the lounge door and absorbs the arrival of her sisters, starts to put the pieces of the puzzle together now her world has shifted slightly once again.

I take The Caulbearer up to the bathroom, sit her on the bathmat and help her to take off her clothes. Her pale body is dotted with spots, with more appearing even as I turn her round and lift her hair from her neck. She is agitated and exhausted until she climbs into the bath and soaks her angry skin. I find a flannel and dip it into the warm water, squeezing it over her shoulders and arms and watching the muscles on her face relax.

I will repeat this activity in a couple of hours, kneel by the bath as calamine lotion soaks into the lavender-infused water. While I am squeezing the flannel over The Caulbearer's skin, The Mermaid will come in telling me she needs a cuddle. She is in between worlds again. She will collapse into my lap and hold onto me tightly in case I am only in her head and liable to drift away. And then The Littlest One will appear at the door, teeth all brushed and clutching a book, while The Whirlwind hops up and down the stairs. I have no idea how I can do The Littlest One's bedtime story, moored as I am by various daughters, so I ask her to read a poem to me, all the while squeezing the water and stroking long mermaid hair. *Read this one all in one breath Mummy* The Littlest One says, holding her book out in front of me. So I do, hundreds of words spilling out of me in one long breath, and I wonder if one day I will dive into the sea, stay deep under the water with burning lungs and reappear miles from the shore.

There is something very intense about this moment. I am the moon, gazing down on my family from high above, watching the mothering and the caring and the juggling, hearing the calm in my voice as my heart flickers fast. And it looks like a lot. It is a lot. But I am enough, with my hands that stroke and my voice that soothes. I must be enough.

On Christmas Eve it becomes apparent that we will not be meeting the children's dad on the beach tomorrow - the Caulbearer is too ill. Our beach trip is postponed, in a year that has seen so many cancellations and disappointments. I have become the mistress of salvaging situations though, and begin to create a space full of lights, flames and treats in our little front room.

The walls are white, floorboards stripped, and the blind sewn by my mum leaks rich flowers and berries across the window like a Tudor banquet. That first summer after he had gone I spent days slapping white paint over the dark, dark grey walls, hoping that a new colour would change me too. Back then I was still completely lost. When I looked in the mirror I saw only shadows of myself that were reflected in other people's eyes, fragments of a woman. I would listen to podcasts as I wiped cobwebs from skirting boards and cleaned brushes, trying out different versions of myself, wondering who might emerge from the wreckage. There was a constant emptiness in my stomach that I can now identify as fear. I have chased it away for the most part now, but it returns intermittently, a kind of post-traumatic terror that I must actively confront so it doesn't swallow me again.

The white paint helped though, faded some of the darkness, and tonight the walls glisten with the reflections of fairy lights and candles, and a log burner that flickers in the gleam of the polished floor. There is a tin of Quality Street, crisps, cheese, carrot sticks, olives, peach juice for the girls and a glass of wine for me. A picnic in the lounge and Little Women on the TV.

A therapist once remarked that my life sounded like Little Women, with all the daughters and the home educating and the singing around the piano, and it felt like the biggest compliment of my life. As I sit cross-legged on a cushion passing crisps to a spotty Caulbearer, Emily Watson is channelling her best Marmee on the screen and telling Jo that she has been angry every day of her life, and this resonates with me so much I feel a leap in my stomach. The concept of endless gentle parenting while fire burns in the belly is my daily lived experience. Marmee describes it with such elegance, makes the act of raising daughters look like such a gift, a fierce woman simmering under the mother. I feel this gift every day, even when I am dragging my feet with exhaustion, eyes gritty and red. The constant contradiction of mothering.

Later that evening, once the dishwasher is stacked and the flames in the log burner are dying, The Whirlwind helps The Littlest One find a carrot for Rudolph, and the girls arrange a mince pie and a glass of milk for Father Christmas. We place the refreshments carefully on the hearth and hope that the fire will have gone out by the time he tries to squeeze down our chimney.

There is more dabbing of calamine onto The Caulbearer's angry little body and I notice a couple of suspicious spots on The Littlest One's back. By Boxing Day she will be covered, her customary bounce will be deflated, and I will give her midnight baths to soothe the itching as hot tears pour from her bush baby eyes. Christmas Eve is calm though, gently fizzing with the hope of heavy stockings lying across legs, and as I pad across the landing towards the bathroom, the Cold Moon hangs in the black night then drifts out of sight, a chalky curve swallowed by the clouds.

On Christmas Day, The Caulbearer is still weak from the pox and reluctant to do much more than cling on to me. Father Christmas has been to visit - The Littlest One has checked by the fire to make sure he has eaten his mince pie and drunk his milk. The cat plays with wrapping paper on my bedroom floor as five of us cuddle up in the bed like a scene from Charlie and the Chocolate Factory. The girls take it in turns to delve into stockings I made when they were born - stretchy pink or red fabric with stitches that are barely holding the seams together after years of Christmas Eve visitations. The younger girls do a festive quiz on Zoom with their dad, six blue eyes staring through a screen at two more.

I always like to wake up in our own house on Christmas Day. It feels like an indication that we have lasted another year, managed not to become any more unstuck. Everything is where it should be, even if it is a little broken. Last Christmas, when The Mermaid was barely out of hospital, she had just moved out of the makeshift bedroom I had made for her in the lounge and back upstairs. I had to walk her to the bathroom as she leaned into me, her legs dragging and aching. Or I would hear a

sliding of cloth against wood, and it would be her, shuffling on her bottom along the landing.

There are no pictures of The Mermaid from last
Christmas, which is unusual. I try to take photos of all of
the girls on special days, and sometimes I send them to
their dad. Perhaps she was feeling particularly self-con-
scious and I understood that. Or maybe I knew that
future me didn't want to remember how poorly she was
or see the nightmares dancing behind her eyes. The nightmares were definitely there. They didn't explode into a
warped reality for another few weeks, but they were lying
dormant, slowly twisting her thoughts and screaming at
her soul. Last Christmas her body was refusing to coop-
erate, and soon her mind would follow. I'm pretty sure
the absence of photos was an act of self-preservation.

If I look further back in time, just after our world caved
in, there are two videos on my phone of The Mermaid in
deep distress. I am ashamed of those videos now, my
thumb hovers over delete whenever I find them, but they
are still there. I had been on a website scrolling through
messages from desperate parents, wondering how they
managed to persuade medical professionals that their
child was exceedingly ill, that someone needed to listen.
And a couple of people on these threads said that they
had filmed their child so that the authorities would believe
them. So one evening I did this, I filmed my daughter
while her eyes were flickering and her limbs were jerking.
I can hear my voice trying to soothe her *please come
upstairs my love*. I am trying to do the right thing - *its ok*

Mummy's here - but at the same time I am making a record of her trauma because my voice is not enough, no one is listening. And my voice is her voice, because she cannot speak in the appointments, she just sits politely in her neat clothes and they look at me like I am mad. *How do you discipline her* (psychologist)? *We need more evidence* (psychiatrist). *Why doesn't she go to school* (everyone)? No one listened.

Maybe I keep the videos on my phone to remind me how bad those days were. There is still a very powerful narrative floating around that threatens to knock me off kilter. No one can see it of course, it's like a will o' the wisp trailing around window frames and pouring poison into my ear. Maybe it will never leave and I will have to keep finding ways to escape it. I feel bad about those videos, but they remind me to keep shouting.

Late December dissolves into a puddle of calamine lotion and chocolate wrappers. I get very little sleep because The Littlest One is absolutely covered from head to toe in chicken pox and needs me constantly. But it doesn't matter about the sleep because we can light the fire, watch films, play games and read books. And as soon as The Littlest One is feeling up to it we wrap up warm and drive to the beach.

Unsurprisingly there is some dissent surrounding a wild winter walk. The wind is fierce and squally showers are flinging themselves against the car windows as we pull up at Seaton Point. Only a few weeks ago some of the beach huts huddling on the cliff top were hurled into the sea by Storm Arwen, and as The Caulbearer clutches my hand and I look down to onto the sand I can see it is covered in seaweed, strips of gnarly bladderwrack lying in great clumps all the way along to the next bay. The Littlest One loves to be outdoors, she is running ahead even as the wind buffets her around. A kestrel hangs in the air above us and darts down towards the ground as we approach. The Mermaid is strong today. She has detailed information about where we are walking and how long for, and her brain can cope as long as we do not divert from the plan. The Whirlwind has no desire to come for a walk with her family, but has promised me she will run a mile in laps around the house in her new running gear. This seems like a reasonable compromise. The Caulbearer, on the other hand, has failed to return to her bouncy self since recovering from chicken pox. She is pale and tinier than usual, and extremely distressed at being brought out for a walk. The wind is too loud and the cold air stings her face, everything is too much. And as I pull her gently along, desperate myself to breathe the fresh salty breeze after more days of confinement, I think to myself *I have been here before.*

In the days to come, as school reopens, this little daughter will not want to return. She will creep into my bed at night, refuse to go to sleep as her breathing quickens until her hand is touching mine. She will pin herself under the duvets in the morning so I have to pull her out to dress her and her fairy hair will stick to flushed cheeks. Her voice, already gentle, will almost entirely disappear and I will spend a lot of time composing emails to the head-teacher. A familiar narrative will grow louder once more, one that suggests I am at fault. And I will wonder why a new year feels so very much like the old one.

But in many ways the new year will be as full of promise as a clear night sky. Perhaps I have been living in the aftermath of the grandest gesture of all, the one where I decided I was worth fighting for. In so many ways, my family looks different from the one I dreamed of, but my life, like all lives, is one of contradiction. The claustrophobia I have experienced in the middle of nowhere could have happened on the busiest street in the world. I have spent years thinking I was trapped by circumstance, feet endlessly itchy, but the claustrophobia was inside my head. Months of confinement to our house, caused by caring for a poorly child and exacerbated by a global disaster, ironically mean that my world has never felt wider. Now that my head belongs only to me once more I have allowed myself to be mesmerised by pockets of beauty that punctuate the day. The school run has become a kind of meditation as we notice again and again the gap between the houses behind the school that frames the waves each morning. The patch of grass next to a bridge where we spot bunnies nibbling in the morning. Gateways where we pull in to watch the sky burning or the sun melting into scrubby fields.

It is hard to overestimate the shame and sadness that has been caused by the fracturing of my family, the total devastation of watching children in pain, the frustration of not being able to explain why it is better to have parents living in different houses, especially when another narrative is so compelling. And though it still hurts a lot to admit it, the heartbreak of failing to continue to grow a love that I wanted to last forever has scarred me. I still can't allow myself to remember too vividly the times when I thought we were invincible. There are memories so precious I daren't write them down in case exposing them to the light destroys them forever.

I grew up being told that I could be anyone, do anything, existing in a bubble of naivety that only popped when I was well into adulthood. I still believe this now, but I didn't see how messy life can be until I left home, and I thought that I wanted this level of protection from reality for my own children. In some ways, my unpreparedness for life, my blinkered optimism, has been my downfall. I can only hope that the challenges my daughters have had to face, the sadness they have seen, will prepare them as they grow older, offer them an extra layer of resilience. Mainly I hope that I have shown them that no one can steal their voices. They might sometimes be drowned out, or become confused when someone twists their truth, or forget who they are and what they want to say. They may wax and wane, shift under other people's gazes, but they are constant.

The Cold Moon is dwindling, a lopsided grin smiling wryly on a turbulent year. The world is spinning, a febrile mass of virus, wild weather and narcissism, but the December skies stretch on forever and I am hopeful.

We climb into the car and drive north across the border, where bricks blush under a low winter sun. The cliffs rise high above a sea reflecting a cloudless sky and a grey seal pup flops onto a pebbled beach. The Mermaid strides ahead like a miracle, dreaming of the moment cold water will wrap itself around her body. The Whirlwind and The Littlest One chatter and trip over stones as I call out to them to keep away from the edge. The Caulbearer stays close to me, but soon she will unfurl and run forwards, and the four of them will move together as one into the sunset, the most beautiful silhouette I have ever seen.

As I walk behind my daughters, my heart is light at the prospect of a new year. A pod of dolphins is heading south towards Northumberland, rainbow arcs catching the low winter light. When I started this journey as a mother on her own, I felt tethered in a strange wild land, missing parts of myself that had developed under the glare of city lights. I thought that living in the middle of nowhere with the huge caring responsibility that is four young daughters meant that I had disappeared. And then when The Mermaid got so poorly and the caring notched up another level I thought my wings had been clipped entirely.

But the way my life has unfolded, sometimes on the edge of what society expects, has required me to be feral in my desire to build a new one, almost as if the wilderness surrounding my home has inhabited me. I will always crave the city - its tempo matches my own - but I also remember the days I stood in the park at the top of the hill with a baby Mermaid in my buggy and couldn't see where the city ended. I remember dreaming of the Yorkshire dales where I had grown up, wanting to breathe air that wouldn't cling to me all day.

Before things began to disintegrate, my husband would often comment on my inability to make my mind up or stay fixed in one place. There would be light and laughter in his blue eyes as he said it, and my restless spirit felt like a good thing. I am still restless now, but perhaps I am learning how to live with itchy feet, a tireless brain. There is safety in my house, my children know it is home. We may not have travelled the whole world together (yet), but our adventures are found on the journeys we make to crescent beaches, secret waterfalls and ancient hills. We are revealed in the stars reflected in our eyes - the grand gestures that shine brighter, and tiny sparks that burn for longer, fizzing and simmering under our gaze.

And always there is the moon. Reclining in the sky, slim and cheeky; an orb rising high above the rooftops; submerged in cloud and felt only in the tides, or stunning the night with its glow. The knowledge that the moon is constant makes me feel small in the very best of ways: not so that I am diminished, but reminding me that the world is vast and unpredictable, and that anything is possible.

Acknowledgements

Twelve Moons has been waxing for several years. When I was newly alone in 2018 I attended an Arvon course that helped me to believe in my words. I owe gratitude to Marina Benjamin, who made me realise I was writing around the real story and encouraged me to dig deeper, and to Cathy Rentzenbrink, whose generous mentoring inspired me to raise my game.

Endless thanks to everyone involved in the MA in Nature and Travel Writing at Bath Spa University, especially Stephen Moss and Gail Simmons. The accessibility of the MA made learning possible for me and opened up my world. My colleagues on the course were not only generous with their creative input but also on a personal level, frequently reaching out during very dark days. Their friendship has been a highlight of the course.

Thank you to Joe Pontin at BBC Countryfile magazine for the opportunity that changed everything.

I'm grateful to Tanya Shadrick for her gentle wisdom. A phone conversation with Tanya when this book was waxing highlighted to me the value of the online writing community, and a fragment of words in this book first appeared in her generous writing project, The Cure For Sleep: Stories From (& Beyond) the Book. Some early words about my Grannie featured in a film I made with Jodie Russi-Red and Naomi Marklew for New Writing North last year, and I have happy memories of recording them on a swinging bench in the gardens of Josephine Butler College at Durham University. Thank you to Tom Stanger at The Pilgrim, who published some early words on Northumberland that grew into Song Moon, and to Sally Saunders at Psychologies for her belief in my work.

I feel lucky to belong to the world's best writing group. Thank you Ilona Bannister, Sarah Gregory, Ali Millar, Nicola Washington and Penny Wincer. These five brilliant women enrich my life every day with their intelligence, humour and kindness.

Thank you to everyone at HarperNorth, especially my editor, Genevieve Pegg. Gen's patience and sensitivity have helped me to manage the challenges involved in writing memoir, and I am fortunate that she is such a fierce champion of my work. I'm grateful too to Alice Murphy-Pyle for her support and advice.

Thank you to my agent, Tim Bates at Peters Fraser and Dunlop, who is calm and pragmatic when I am emotional and impulsive. I am glad to have him on my team. Also Daisy Chandley, who is always efficient and reassuring. I have been delighted to have the opportunity to work with Emma Finnigan on the publicity for Twelve Moons, so huge thanks to her as well.

So many friends have held me over the last few years. I feel lucky that my daughters and I have been surrounded by love and generosity even when we have been isolated. Special thanks to Lotte, who never stops believing in me, to Sue for her advice and love, and to Bunny for the expertise and solidarity. Thank you to my local friends: Shelly, who brings me coffee when I go into hiding; Louise, who picked me up from the kitchen floor and

Acknowledgements

helped me to keep going; Sonia, who listened to me while I cried quietly in my front garden so the children didn't hear; Helen, for the conversations while we run and swim; and Lyn, who is so kind to my girls and has played endless silly games with them so that I can get out of the house for an hour.

Huge thanks to Mum and Dad, who told me to pursue my dreams when they seemed impossible and listened to my voice when other narratives were louder. Thank you to my brothers, Andy (the real writer in the family) and Greg, and to my sister, Cath, who is always there despite the sea between us.

Finally, thank you most of all to my four daughters, who are generous, supportive and inspirational, and who show me every day what it means to be brave. I love you.